THE ART THERAPY SOURCEBOOK

CATHY A. MALCHIODI, ATR, LPCC

McGraw·Hill

New York   Chicago   San Francisco   Lisbon   London   Madrid   Mexico City
Milan   New Delhi   San Juan   Seoul   Singapore   Sydney   Toronto

Library of Congress Cataloging-in-Publication Data

Malchiodi, Cathy A.
    The art therapy sourcebook / Cathy A. Malchiodi.—2nd ed.
       p.   cm.
    Includes bibliographical references and index.
    ISBN 0-07-146827-7
    1. Art therapy.   I. Title.

    RC489.A7M345   2007
    616.89′1656—dc22   2006001325

11 12 13 14 15   DOC/DOC 1 9 8 7 6 5 4 3

ISBN-13: 978-0-07-146827-5
ISBN-10:   0-07-146827-7

McGraw-Hill books are available at special quantity discounts to use as premiums and sales promotions, or for use in corporate training programs. For more information, please write to the Director of Special Sales, Professional Publishing, McGraw-Hill, Two Penn Plaza, New York, NY 10121-2298. Or contact your local bookstore.

This book is printed on acid-free paper.

In memory of Gita Akots

Contents

Acknowledgments

ALTHOUGH THE AUTHOR'S name appears on the cover of a book, the actual writing that goes into it is always a collaborative process that involves family, friends, and colleagues and a little luck along the way. In writing the original sourcebook and this revised edition, I was helped by many friends and colleagues in ways that are difficult to quantify or define, but without their support this book would not have become a reality. Some helped by simply listening to me think out loud for endless hours on the phone. Others read and responded to perpetual e-mails. And all have supported my work as an art therapist, artist, and writer. Thanks to (in alphabetical order) Pat Allen, Mariagnese Cattaneo, Carol Thayer Cox, Cay Drachnik, Lynn Kapitan, Frances Kaplan, Jessica Kingsley, Don Jones, Shaun McNiff, Shirley Riley, Anna Riley-Hiscox, Judy Rubin, Diane Safran, Bernie Siegel, Rochelle Serwator, Susan Spaniol, Bill Steele, Bobbi Stoll, Kay Stovall, Janis Timm-Bottos, Lori Vance, Ewa Wasilewska, and Barbara Wheeler.

Thanks also to all the individuals whom I have been privileged to work with in my art therapy practice, groups, and workshops and who shared their stories and images for this book. They continually teach me why art making restores, repairs, transforms, and heals.

Last, thanks to my patient husband, David Barker, without whom this book would not have been possible.

Introduction

THE LANGUAGE OF visual art—colors, shapes, lines, and images—speaks to us in ways that words cannot. Art therapy is a modality that uses the nonverbal language of art for personal growth, insight, and transformation and is a means of connecting what is inside us—our thoughts, feelings, and perceptions—with outer realities and life experiences. It is based on the belief that images can help us understand who we are and enhance life through self-expression.

While the field of art therapy is relatively new, the idea that art making can be a form of therapy is very old, and art making is one of the most ancient forms of healing. The visual arts—drawing, painting, and sculpture—are powerful and effective forms of communication that have been used to convey humanity's collective history, ideas, feelings, dreams, and aspirations. Art has always been used to chronicle and portray a wide range of emotions and experiences, from profound joy to the deepest sorrow, from triumph to trauma. Since our earliest recorded history, art has also served as a means of reparation, rehabilitation, and transformation and has been used to restore physical, psychological, and spiritual well-being.

In recent years, we have rediscovered the benefits of art making for personal growth, self-expression, transformation, and wellness. Many people have found that art making can be soothing and stress reducing, a way to transcend troubling circumstances or life's problems. Others have experienced how imagery can help people to solve problems, release powerful or distressing emotions, and recover from traumatic losses or experiences and can alleviate pain or other physical symptoms. You yourself may already be using art as a form of therapy and may paint, draw, or sculpt for relaxation, gratification, and self-expression.

In response to this recognition that art can help people to authentically express themselves, release powerful emotions, and transcend trauma and can enhance health and well-being, the field of art therapy has grown and expanded since the 1970s, becoming a recognized form of treatment in health and medicine. Art therapy is based on the idea that the creative process of art making is healing and life enhancing and that it is a potent form of communication. It utilizes the creative process, which exists within every individual, to promote growth, self-expression, emotional reparation, conflict resolution, and transformation. Through art making as therapy you may find relief from overwhelming emotions, crises, or trauma; discover insights about yourself; achieve an increased sense of well-being; enrich your daily life; or experience personal change. It is a way to make sense of that which is painful, to create personal meaning, to enhance wellness, and to become whole.

The revised edition of this book will provide you with a comprehensive and contemporary overview of the field of art therapy and explain the power of art making for personal growth, insight, and transformation. It will tell you what art therapy is, where it came from, and why it is a powerful way of knowing yourself and is recognized by psychology, mental health counseling, and medicine as an important form of healing. It will also familiarize you with some of the many ways art making as therapy can help you authentically express yourself and confront and resolve trauma or loss, as well as reduce your level of stress and enhance your health and well-being.

Because art therapy is an action-oriented, experiential modality for self-exploration and growth, it is important that you experience it not only through reading this book but also through your own art making. What I have described about art therapy will be more meaningful if you become an active participant in learning about art's healing potential through expressing yourself in the simple drawing, painting, and collage exercises presented throughout this book. What I have learned about the therapeutic benefits of art making has partially come from reading about and studying the field of art therapy and through my own work as an artist. My personal experiences of art making as therapy have shown me its transformative and reparative qualities.

I have also learned from others—clients, artists, students, and colleagues—why art is restorative and healing; many of their stories are described throughout this book. In almost three decades of working as an art therapist with abused or traumatized children, people with serious illnesses, and families experiencing trauma or loss and through teaching thousands of people in art therapy workshops and studios, I have been repeatedly taught about important connections between the creative process of image making and health. These experiences have proven to me that art is a potent and effective means of self-expression available to people of all ages and capabilities, that everyone can benefit from art's ability to repair and restore, and that art making as therapy can play a vital role in health, healing, and wholeness.

1

What Is Art Therapy?

Art can be said to be—and can be used as—the externalized map of our interior self.

PETER LONDON, NO MORE SECONDHAND ART

AT ONE TIME or another we all have experienced the creative and personally enriching potential of art. As a child, you probably found enjoyment in making crayon drawings, cut-paper collages, sand castles, or handprints in clay. As an adult, you may not consider yourself to be creative or an artist, but you still may have experienced some therapeutic aspects of art in your daily life. You may paint or take photographs as a hobby, enjoying the process of creation and recognizing that creative activities help relieve stress. You may keep a drawing diary, sketching your dreams, noting symbols, and thinking about their meanings. You may scribble lines on the corner of your notepad on your desk, finding that it helps you think more clearly and relax. All of these activities are ways to soothe yourself, release stress and tension, give enjoyment and pleasure, and transcend troubling feelings. They are methods of self-expression that change your state of being and tap your intuitive and creative powers.

Although you have experienced some of art making's therapeutic powers, you still may not think of art as related to therapy. Depending on your personal definition of art, you may think of it as something used as decoration, entertainment, or novelty or only as those paintings and sculptures that are exhibited in museums and galleries. You may see art as only child's play or perhaps as a diversion or hobby. While art is sometimes difficult to define, you would probably agree that art enhances your existence, but you may not be fully aware of all the ways that art can be life enhancing.

While art can serve as decoration or hang in a museum, there are other purposes for art, ones that are connected to self-understanding, a search for meaning, personal growth, self-empowerment, and healing. Many of us have lost contact with these purposes or have not realized that art is more than novelty or ornamentation. Drawing, painting, sculpture, and other art forms are powerful and effective forms of communication, and cultures through the ages have been defined and understood through their art. While art has been used to record human history, it has also incorporated our ideas, feelings, dreams, and aspirations. Art chronicles and conveys a wide range of emotions, from profound joy to the deepest sorrow, from triumph to trauma. In this sense, art has served as a way of understanding, making sense, and clarifying inner experiences without words.

Art therapy has grown from this concept that art images can help us to understand who we are, to express feelings and ideas that words cannot, and to enhance life through self-expression. It is accepted and widely recognized as a viable treatment method and a modality for self-understanding, emotional change, and personal growth.

Art + Therapy = ?

People new to art therapy are often confused about just what the term *art therapy* means. While it was coined to describe the use of art expression in therapy, it frequently generates some unusual assumptions. Over the years, I have heard many interesting impressions of what art therapy might be, some of which are quite humorous. I once was asked if art therapy is only for "sick" or "disturbed" artists, providing a special treatment for curing their depressions, anxieties, or creative blocks. I was recently asked if art therapy could help improve one's drawing and painting abilities. Another person inquired if I worked with paintings and sculptures that had "problems." Apparently, he imagined that art therapy could make "bad" paintings and sculptures look better! It is easy to understand that the term *art therapy* can be confusing when first encountered and especially if one has not had any personal experience with it.

There are several reasons why art therapy is not easily understood. First, art therapy is practiced with a wide range of people. The use of art therapy has been documented with a variety of populations including children, adolescents, adults, and the elderly; people with addictions; individuals with serious and sometimes terminal illnesses; war veterans; people with disabilities; families experiencing difficulties; prisoners; and individuals experiencing a wide spectrum of emotional disorders. You may have heard of art therapy being used with children who have been traumatized by abuse, with troubled families to explore their problems, or with disabled older adults in nursing homes. You may know of a psychologist who asks his or her patients to make drawings as part of their therapy or an expressive therapist who uses art to help people deal with chronic pain or other symptoms. You may have read in the newspaper about an artist who works with paraplegics, helping them paint, or about a therapist who has created an art studio for disabled adults. There may be an art therapist who works in your local school system with children with learning or developmental problems or one who works at the medical center in your community with children and adults with cancer. These are all common examples of where art therapy is used, demonstrating the vast diversity of the field.

Another reason why many people are confused about art therapy comes from the experiential nature of art itself. Art therapy is a dynamic therapy, requiring one to participate in one's own treatment, in this case through art making. Therefore, truly understanding art therapy requires firsthand experience.

The combination of the words *art* and *therapy* also can be confusing. Art therapist and psychologist Judith Rubin coined the phrase that opens this section: Art + Therapy = ? This formula conveys the equation that makes up art therapy—the blending of art and therapy. Art therapy is essentially the marriage of two disciplines: art and psychology. Aspects of the visual arts, the creative process, human development, behavior, personality, and mental health, among others, are important to the definition and scope of art therapy. Art therapy brings together all of these disciplines, making it difficult to understand at first glance.

Finally, as strange as it sounds, some of the confusion about art therapy may come from art therapists themselves. When you ask art therapists what they do, each offers many examples, in part because art therapy is practiced with a variety of populations. To make matters even more perplexing, there is even some disagreement within the professional field about how to define art therapy. Because there are so many definitions of art therapy, the next several sections of this chapter cover the ideas that have shaped the field and have distinguished art therapy from other modalities that have been used to enhance health and well-being.

Drawing from Within

There once was a popular phrase among many art therapists: art therapy—draw from within. This is a good elementary definition of art therapy and helps to distinguish it from other ways in which art is used. While an art therapy session may look like an art class on the surface, the goals and purposes are different. For example, in a typical studio art class you might be asked to draw a model, paint a composition from a still life, or sketch what you see on a nature walk in the forest. You are usually asked to draw something you see and to work at rendering it with accurate proportions, shading, and color, emphasizing technical skills and craftsmanship.

Art therapist Don Jones, one of the founders of the field of art therapy, precisely captures the essence of "drawing from within" in the self-portrait painting *Who, What, Where, How?* (Figure 1.1). Jones depicts himself looking down at a pool of water and imagining his own reflection. His closed eyes emphasize the inner experience of knowing oneself through art and imagination.

Art therapy asks you to explore your inner experience—your feelings, perceptions, and imagination. While art therapy may involve learning skills or art techniques, the emphasis is generally first on developing and expressing images that come from inside the person, rather than those he or she sees in the outside world. And while some traditional art classes may ask you to paint or draw from

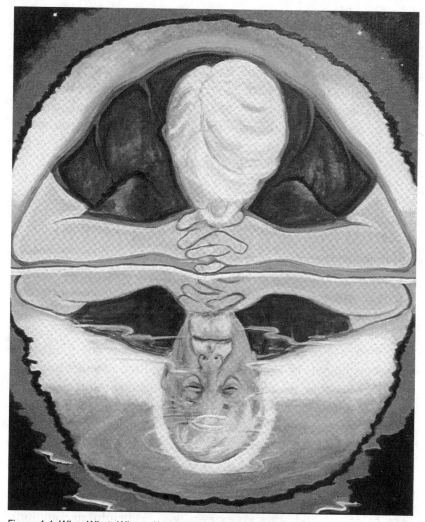

Figure 1.1 *Who, What, Where, How?*, by art therapist Don Jones
(Reprinted with permission of the artist)

your imagination, in art therapy, your inner world of images, feelings, thoughts, and ideas is consistently important and primary to the experience.

Therapy comes from the Greek word *therapeia*, which means "to be attentive to." This meaning underscores the art therapy process in two ways. In most cases, a skilled professional attends to the individual who is making the art. This person's guidance is key to the therapeutic process. This supportive relationship is necessary to guide the art-making experience and to help the individual find meaning through it along the way.

The other important aspect is the attendance of the individual to his or her own personal process of making art and to giving the art product personal meaning—that is, finding a story, description, or meaning for the art. Very few therapies depend as much on the active participation of the individual.

Art + Therapy = Process + Product

Although art therapists have generated many specific definitions of art therapy, most of them fall into one of two general categories. The first involves a belief in the inherent healing power of the creative process of art making. This view embraces the idea that the process of making art is therapeutic; this process is sometimes referred to as art as therapy. Art making is seen as an opportunity to express oneself imaginatively, authentically, and spontaneously, an experience that, over time, can lead to personal fulfillment, emotional reparation, and transformation. This view also holds that the creative process, in and of itself, can be a health-enhancing and growth-producing experience.

The second definition of art therapy is based on the idea that art is a means of symbolic communication. This approach, often referred to as art psychotherapy, emphasizes the products—drawings, paintings, and other art expressions—as helpful in communicating issues, emotions, and conflicts. Psychotherapy is essential to this approach, and the art image becomes significant in enhancing verbal exchange between the person and the therapist and in achieving insight. With therapeutic guidance and support, art can facilitate new understandings and insights. It can help people to resolve conflicts, solve problems, and formulate new perceptions that in turn lead to positive changes, growth, and healing.

In reality, most therapists who practice art therapy integrate both art as therapy and art psychotherapy into their work in varying degrees. In other words, both the idea that art making can be a healing process and that art products communicate information relevant to therapy are important. Therapists may emphasize one area over another, depending on their own philosophy and the person's needs and goals in art therapy.

What About Interpretation?

Many people wonder if art therapy is purely about interpreting the content of art expressions. On occasion, I am confronted by a person who wants me to analyze his or her paintings or another therapist who wants to know if I can tell from a child's drawing whether that child has been abused or traumatized. Images are forms of nonverbal communication, and you naturally may wonder if they contain any hidden meanings or if it is possible to interpret their content. Many people who participate in art therapy are also interested in finding out more about what their images mean.

Some of people's curiosity about interpreting art comes from their familiarity with psychological tests designed to evaluate personality. You may know about the Rorschach test, which involves responding to ink-blot images, or you may have heard that drawings are occasionally used by psychologists as aids to diagnosis. Since art therapy does involve image making, it is natural to assume that it may involve interpreting art for the purpose of assessment or diagnosis.

To some extent, art therapists are interested in the meaning of people's paintings, drawings, and other types of artwork and are intrigued by images and symbols. A great deal of research is being conducted to determine if there are recurring symbols, artistic content, and styles of drawing that may be connected to emotional disorders, trauma, physical illness, or neurological problems. For example, art therapists have researched what types of content recur in the art expressions of adults who have been diagnosed with dissociative disorders and severe childhood trauma. Many therapists have explored the symbolic and structural aspects of mandala (circle) drawings to see if there are any connections between images and colors and certain psychological or physical conditions. Psychologists, clinical counselors, art therapists, and others are exploring what simple human figure drawings can reveal about personality, development, trauma, and neurological symptoms, among other things. This type of work focuses more on the use of art expressions in assessment rather than in personal growth or self-understanding.

While there is a fascination with the meaning of art made in therapy, most art therapists are more interested in helping the person who makes the art come up with his or her own interpretation. Asking people to reflect on their work is an important part of the art therapy process for several reasons. First, while there seems to be some universal symbols in art expression, the way you express yourself through art is often very personal. You bring your own unique background to art making, including previous life experiences, cultural influences, and personal perspectives. Your individual experience with art making also affects how you convey your feelings, thoughts, and ideas through art. In art therapy, however, this aspect is extremely helpful because the person who creates the art determines what the image means. These responses are all part of the therapeutic process and are as personal and individual as the art itself.

Also, the meaning of an art image is truly in the eye of the beholder. If you and I look at the same painting, we are both likely to see slightly different aspects and to have a completely different interpretation of what the image is about. If I look at a painting that a person has made in art therapy without consulting the person about its meaning, I probably will impose my own meaning on the piece. We naturally have a tendency to project or transfer our beliefs, impressions, ideas, and feelings onto images we see. Finally, art expressions can also change meanings over time. That is, if you look at a drawing or painting several weeks from now, you may see new aspects and have new reactions and responses to what you see. This is part of the magic of art but also part of its mystery when it comes to establishing a singular meaning for a drawing, painting, or sculpture.

Why Art Therapy Helps

While art can be used to achieve some degree of understanding of the person who makes it, the process of art therapy and its potential to help people grow, rehabilitate, and heal also comes from the actual making of art. Helping people understand their art expressions can certainly be part of art therapy, but the process of making art is equally important. Art therapy is a modality with special qualities for reparation, transformation, and self-exploration.

Visual Thinking

Visual thinking is our ability and tendency to organize our feelings, thoughts, and perceptions about the world around us through images. It pervades everything we do, from planning our day to dreaming at night. We often use visual references to describe our perceptions of people and things we experience in our everyday lives. Most of us are familiar with the cliché "A picture is worth a thousand words" or sayings about colors, such as "She was green with envy," "I have the blues," or "He looks at the world through rose-colored glasses." We designate and characterize the world with visual descriptions; we think in images, often using them to represent thoughts and feelings.

Sigmund Freud, considered to be the father of modern psychology, observed that dreams, feelings, and thoughts are experienced predominantly in visual form. He concluded that his patients' frustrations in describing their dreams might be alleviated if they could draw them. Freud also realized that art is closer to the unconscious because our visual perceptions predate our capacity for verbal expression. Images are part of our earliest experiences, and many of our preverbal thoughts are in images. Even as adults, while we may remember an event, a place, or a person through senses such as sound or smell, we are also likely to have a mental image of the experience.

Carl Jung, known for his interest in visual symbols in dreams and art, also noted the importance of images in therapy. He observed that by allowing a mood or problem to become personified or by representing it as an image through dreams or art, we can begin to understand it more clearly and deeply and to experience the emotions that are contained within it. Jung's philosophy has influenced the field of psychotherapy, which has relied heavily on the images of memories and dreams and their connection to feelings in helping people work through emotional conflicts and problems.

More recently, researchers have discovered that traumatic experiences often become encoded in the mind in the form of images. That is, when we experience traumatic events such as violent acts or catastrophes, our minds may take them in just like a camera taking a photograph. It seems only natural that these memories would first emerge in the form of images. Visual art may offer a unique way to express traumatic images, bringing them to consciousness in a less threatening way.

Although I have worked with hundreds of children and adults who have been traumatized, one case in particular demonstrates how experiences of severe trauma may return in the form of images, even before words are available to describe them. A few years ago a young woman, Carla, came to see me with a knapsack of sketchbooks filled with drawings she had created over the last several months. Carla said that she had never been interested in art until recently. She felt compelled each day to make drawings of images, some from her dreams and others from her imagination (Figures 1.2 and 1.3). The content of these images troubled her, and she thought that perhaps sharing them with an art therapist might help her understand them. The majority of the drawings contained what were obviously violent and painful scenes. The style of the draw-

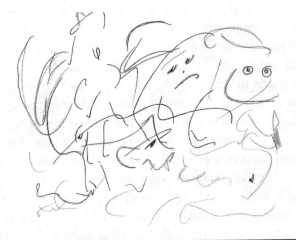

Figure 1.2 *Our Personalities*, a pencil and felt-tip pen drawing depicting multiple personalities, by Carla   *(Reprinted with permission of the artist)*

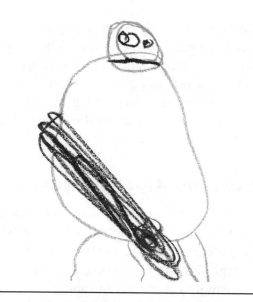

Figure 1.3 A crayon drawing by Carla of her abusive father
(Reprinted with permission of the artist)

ings was curious. While some of them looked like images created by an adult, most could easily be mistaken as the drawings of a young child.

In the months that followed, I worked with Carla to help her determine the meaning of her images and to discover why she was compelled to put these images on paper. Through artwork and sessions with a hypnotherapist, we discovered that Carla had suffered severe abuse as a child and was now struggling with dissociative identity disorder (formerly known as multiple personality disorder) as a result. Through art expression she was able to uncover the memories of her abuse and begin the long process of understanding and integrating experiences from which she had dissociated herself, experiences too painful to speak of out loud. Art images also became a way for Carla and me to begin to unravel and identify the multiple personalities that she developed to cope with the severe trauma to which she was subjected by her father during the early years of her life.

The visual language of art making is a less familiar way of communicating and is therefore less controllable. For Carla, art was a safe way to express complex and difficult life experiences; words did not come easily to her. In contrast, words can be a way of avoiding or disguising the expression of true feelings for some people. A nonverbal form of communication such as art can be a window to feelings and thoughts that might not be accessible through language. This quality of art making can open avenues to emotions and ideas that have remained unknown and unconscious.

Expressing What Words Cannot

At one time or another, we all have found that some experiences and feelings are difficult or impossible to express in words. In art therapy, people are encouraged to express what they cannot say with words through drawings, paintings, or other art forms. In Carla's case, her memories of trauma and abuse were so painful that she could initially only express them through drawings. Her drawings served as a way to communicate what had happened to her before she could consciously accept the reality of her childhood experiences. In her case, art helped her to recall childhood memories and express feelings and thoughts not immediately obvious or accessible through words.

Because art expression is not a linear process and need not obey the rules of language, such as syntax, grammar, logic, and correct spelling, it can express many complexities simultaneously. Art therapist Harriet Wadeson calls this art's spatial matrix: the ability of art to communicate relationships using shape, color, and line. For example, explaining the relationships between one's family members may be difficult; in a drawing of the relationships between family members, different times, places, and connections between family members can be easily depicted in the same drawing or painting. What might take paragraphs of words to describe can be expressed much more readily through a single drawing. Ambiguous, confusing, or even contradictory elements can also be put into the same drawing or painting, because art, unlike language, has no rules about structure or organization. This ability of art to contain paradoxical elements helps people integrate and synthesize conflicting feelings and experiences.

Art therapy can be particularly useful with young children. Children do not have extensive vocabularies for describing their feelings and experiences, but they are generally comfortable with art as a natural way to communicate. In recent studies, children who express crises or emotionally laden events through drawing are able to verbally recollect and relate more details about their experiences than through talking alone. The terrorist attacks of September 11, 2001, demonstrated that children were eager to use art to recall what they saw and to symbolize their fears, worries, and questions about what happened (Figure 1.4). While many children saw the events on television and did not experience the World Trade Center or Pentagon disasters firsthand, art allowed them to make sense of their experiences without words.

Sensory Experience

Art making is a hands-on activity—it involves constructing, arranging, mixing, touching, molding, gluing, drawing, stapling, painting, forming, and other tangible experiences. Drawing, painting, and

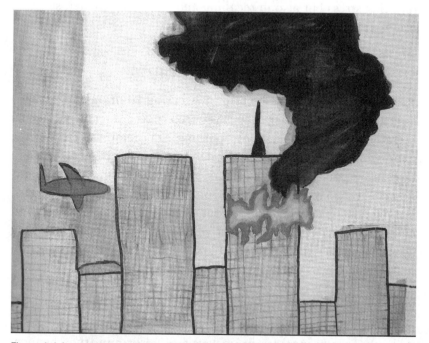

Figure 1.4 An untitled painting by Ryan Sweeney, age fifteen, in response to the terrorist attacks of September 11, 2001 *(Reprinted from* The Day Our World Changed *© 2002 with permission of NYU Child Study Center and Museum of the City of New York)*

sculpting are also psychomotor experiences; that is, they are sensory in nature because they include vision, touch, movement, sound, and other senses, depending on the media used. As children, we learn through our senses—through scribbling on paper, play, and pretend. These experiences, according to psychologist Eugene Gendlin, involve a "felt sense," a bodily awareness of a situation, a person, or an event. In addition to thought, felt sense is a way of making meaning that helps us understand and appreciate the world around us.

The sensory qualities of art making often provide a way for us to tap into our emotions and perceptions more easily than we would with words alone. In cases of emotional trauma, loss, or abuse, art making offers a way to reintegrate complex emotions that are expressed through the senses. Because the tactile aspects of art materials—for example, working with clay, pastels, or paints—can be self-soothing and relaxing, art making also may assist the process of emotional reparation and healing. As you will read in Chapter 7, the sensory qualities of art expression are helpful not only in reducing stress but also in recalling and reframing the felt sense of traumatic memories, grief, and loss.

Emotional Release

Art therapy can also be helpful in releasing emotions. In psychological terms, this experience is referred to as catharsis. *Catharsis* literally means "cleansing" or "purging"; in therapy it refers to the expression and discharge of strong emotions for relief. Making a drawing, a painting, a sculpture, or another art form can be cathartic in that it may provide relief from painful or troubling feelings. For many people, being able to contain their ideas, experiences, and emotions in art can have a positive effect, and for others, talking about what they have portrayed in their images, particularly traumatic experiences or feelings, is cathartic.

The actual process of art making can also alleviate emotional stress and anxiety by creating a physiological response of relaxation or by altering mood. For example, it is known that creative activity can actually increase brain levels of serotonin, the chemical linked to depression. Other people experience art as a form of meditation, finding inner peace and calm through art expression. The repetitive, self-soothing qualities of painting, drawing, or working with clay may induce the "relaxation response," a reduction in heart rate and respiration related to stress reduction.

Creating a Product

In *What Is Art For?* Ellen Dissanayake notes that art making involves our natural interest in creating things with our hands and making things that are special or unique. Art has been used throughout history to embellish and decorate, ways of "making special," which are genuine human proclivities and needs. Some people create something extraordinary or unique through painting or sculpting; others dress in special clothes for important occasions or cook special meals to commemorate an event. These are visual ways of "making special" and are fundamental to human behavior.

Art therapy is perhaps one of few therapies in which you create a tangible product. It offers an opportunity to create something lasting that records meanings, experiences, and feelings. This permanent quality found in art is a distinct benefit because it documents in a concrete manner ideas and perceptions that can be reviewed at a later time and compared with other images. Reviewing art expressions created during several weeks or months allows one to see changes and patterns in thoughts, feelings, events, and themes over time.

Although the creative process and symbolic communication are two fundamental aspects of art therapy, there are several different aspects of the art therapy process that can be considered therapeutic. In its simplest sense, art making is an activity that can generate self-esteem, encourage risk taking and experimentation, teach new skills, and enrich one's life. While this dimension of art therapy may seem like mere recreation, the process of creativity—making something with one's own hands and realizing that one can make something unique—is a powerful experience with undeniable therapeutic benefits. There is something personally meaningful and authentic about creating with one's hands and from one's imagination. Making art touches many different parts of ourselves. It may evoke positive past experiences of drawing or painting as a child or a sense of pride and accomplishment in forming a clay sculpture or arranging images to make a collage.

Creating Art Enhances Life

History shows us that individuals under great stress have been known to make art as a way to express and transform inner conflicts. The creative work of Vincent van Gogh and other well-known visual artists attests to this need. Throughout history, artists have used their art to explore human suffering, to find meaning for their emotional struggles, and to seek transcendence.

Psychologist Abraham Maslow suggested that when people's basic needs—food, shelter, and security—are satisfied, they show a strong drive toward self-expression. Even when deprived of basic necessities, some humans still strive to express themselves through the arts. Despite the constant shelling and sniper fire in Sarajevo in the early 1990s, people continued to express themselves through art. They held concerts, maintained orchestras and choirs, and, at one point, turned a destroyed theater into an exhibition space for art created out of materials from the city's destruction. This illustrates that our drive to express ourselves through art is a powerful and compelling human need.

While art may help us express fear, anxiety, and other stressful emotions, it also touches the soul or spirit. While family, work, and other parts of life may fulfill us, creative experiences with art making can help us express or contact parts of ourselves that other activities and interactions cannot. The story of the people of Sarajevo is a moving example of how art helps us transcend daily life and brings wholeness and personal satisfaction to our lives even though we lack basic needs and safety and are surrounded by destruction and devastation.

Art therapist Bruce Moon believes that art making serves an existential purpose, helping us make sense of a world that seems filled with boredom, dysfunctional relationships, abuse, addictions, and purposelessness. In this sense, art making can help people overcome their feelings of existential emptiness and loss of soul. By making art and using our imaginations, we may find relief from fears, anxiety, and depression and discover new meaning in our lives.

Psychologist Rollo May notes that grace, harmony, beauty, and balance are part of the many qualities of visual art. He observes that art can provide transcendence, allowing people to envision and imagine new possibilities through visual expression and to experience themselves in new ways. The creative process is conducive to individuation, the process of reaching one's full potential, and offers the opportunity for growth and change.

Finally, art making is an enjoyable activity, one that enlivens, energizes, and gives pleasure. People are generally more lively and playful during art making and more communicative with others after finishing the activity. Making art is believed to help one become more flexible, to self-actualize, and to tap creative problem solving and intuition. Through art making, one can also experiment with new ideas, new ways of expression, and new ways of seeing. Finding joy, playing, creating, and communicating in a meaningful way are necessary for psychological, physical, and spiritual health, and making art provides these experiences.

Creating Relationships

Finally, while making art on one's own can be a relaxing, emotionally fulfilling, and self-repairing experience, art therapy's effectiveness capitalizes on the relationship between the art maker and the therapist. In all forms of therapy, the presence of a facilitator or witness is central to healing, reparation, and recovery. An authentic relationship with a therapist, along with the completion of satisfying work (an art product), enhances the potential of art making as a form of treatment. In an art therapy session, the therapist may serve as a supportive guide to a client's exploration of art materials, help an individual examine the content and meaning of images, or provide an empathetic response to the art maker's creative expressions. For many individuals, self-expression in the presence of a helping professional can be an important encounter because the therapist provides encouragement, motivation, acceptance, and positive affirmation that encourage personal growth and self-esteem.

As you will read in Chapter 9, making art in groups emphasizes a unique way of exploring relationships with others. If you have ever taken a studio art course, you probably know that working in the presence of other people stimulates new ideas and creative juices and naturally generates interaction, communication, and exchange. While painting, drawing, or constructing in a group, you have the benefit of seeing the work of other people, receiving responses to your own work, and experiencing the collective energy of a community of art makers. According to art therapist Shaun McNiff, creating art with others or within a group opens up possibilities for personal transformation through sharing your art products and influencing and inspiring the creative potential of other art makers.

Art Making Is Possible for Everyone

A common misconception about art therapy is that you need to have artistic talent to benefit from it. Some people worry that if they do not make technically correct art, art therapy will not be successful or they somehow will have failed. On the contrary, making art in art therapy does not require that you have artistic training. Drawing, painting, and a variety of other art forms are simple methods of expression easily available to almost everyone, regardless of age or abilities. Art making is also a normalizing experience; that is, everyone has the ability to be creative through art.

The philosophy of art therapy embraces the idea that all art expression is acceptable. The purpose is not to make great art. Nevertheless, people still ask me if what they are doing is art therapy, if they are making art or simply experiencing therapy through drawing, painting, or another modality. To define the term *art* is nearly impossible. Scholars, artists, and art historians have pondered the question "What is art?" for hundreds of years without any consensus. Some believe that what results from art therapy is not art because images are created for purposes other than fine art. Throughout the history of art, however, there has been an overlap between art created as fine art or decoration and art made to express views of the artist's inner world.

Perhaps making "great" art is not possible for everyone, but it is possible for most people to be creative and to find art making personally fulfilling. It may be helpful to know that people who have considered themselves to be nonartists have discovered, often accidentally, that art making can be an enriching experience despite their lack of training. One such person is Elizabeth Layton, also known as Grandma Layton, who considered herself to be a nonartist and who came upon drawing as a way to help her recover from thirty years of manic-depressive illness. According to Layton, electroshock treatments, lithium, and psychotherapy failed to bring her any lasting relief from her condition. Following the death of her son in 1976 when she was sixty-seven, Layton took her sister's suggestion and enrolled in a drawing class in a nearby college. The only class available at that time was one in contour drawing. Contour drawings are line drawings created from looking at the object or person one is drawing, rather than looking at the paper on which one is drawing. These drawings, for this reason, often appear distorted but rich in personality and detail.

Layton came to contour drawing having never made art. The course instructor told her that if she had no subject to draw, she should simply draw herself. Layton took this advice and began creating a series of drawings that depicted every wrinkle, age spot, and aspect of her elderly body (Figure 1.5). But other ideas emerged in her work: concerns about society's treatment of the elderly, her own

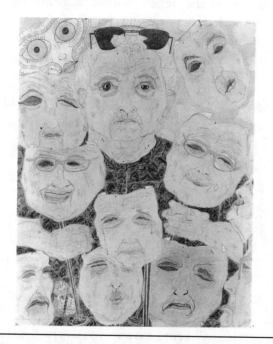

Figure 1.5 *Masks*, a pencil and crayon drawing by Elizabeth Layton. About the piece, Layton said, "What I had in mind was all these emotions you have through your life. There are muscles in your face and each one reacts to every emotion. Say you're happy for a minute, and you put on that mask, and that's going to make an indentation in these muscles to a certain extent. I think it's the various emotions you have had that causes the lines and wrinkles in your face."   *(Reprinted with permission of Don Lambert)*

struggles with aging, and her experience with depression, grief, and loss (Figure 1.6). By confronting and expressing her thoughts, feelings, and perceptions through drawing, she began to feel her depression lift.

Grandma Layton believed that contour drawing had changed her life and alleviated her condition. She later concluded that in addition to the process of drawing, it was the discovery of meaning in each of her drawings that led to her healing. Just as artists often reflect on the content of their images, Layton experienced self-understanding through her art. While creating the images helped her experience catharsis of her intense emotional pain, her written commentaries about her drawings helped her identify the meaning of her portraits and put closure on experiences and feelings that had troubled her throughout her life.

Grandma Layton also began to share more and more of her life story, not only through her drawings but also with artist Don Lambert and art therapist Robert Ault. Layton's conversations with them deepened her understanding of her work and her emotional heal-

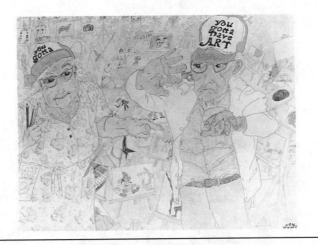

Figure 1.6 *You Gotta Have Art*, a pencil and crayon drawing by Elizabeth Layton. "Art does so much for me I want everyone to try it. If you get tired of my ranting do like Glenn does—duck. My sister Carolyn kept coaxing me to try art, like her husband persuaded her to paint. Daughter Kay even brought me art assignments to do—a child's movie screen in a shoebox, nursery rhymes to illustrate. So, timidly I ventured out into the world of art, enrolled in basic drawing, and discovered CONTOUR!" *(Reprinted with permission of Don Lambert)*

ing. Her drawings have since been appreciated by people throughout the United States and the rest of the world.

Layton never sold any of her drawings, fearing the magic of the process would disappear. She did give many of the more than one thousand drawings she created to family, friends, and charity. Layton's work demonstrates that creativity is important throughout the life span and that feelings need to be expressed, whether through art or other means, in order to be resolved.

Art as a Way of Knowing

For Layton, drawing was more than a means of communicating what was difficult to say with words; it was also a way of knowing her true self. Through art she was able to express profound grief and loss and to understand the emotional distress and depression she experienced for more than three decades. Layton found that art making eventually helped her discover and create a meaning for her life.

In *Art Is a Way of Knowing*, Pat Allen writes that in addition to teaching us what it is to be human and alive, art is also "a way of knowing what we actually believe." In making a drawing or painting, we begin the process of exploring our beliefs. We may find the reason for pain or depression or identify sources of joy and creative potential. Art inevitably tells our personal stories in all their dimensions: our feelings, thoughts, experiences, values, and beliefs. In the process of making these visible through art, we are offered a way to know ourselves from a new perspective and an opportunity to transform that perspective.

Art + Therapy = Powerful Healing

Like most art therapists, I have my own personal definition of what art therapy is and how it works. This definition is a hybrid of the ideas previously mentioned. I believe that my role as an art therapist is to help people explore and express themselves authentically through art. Through this process, people may find relief from overwhelming emotions, crises, or trauma. They may discover insights about themselves, increase their sense of well-being, enrich their daily lives through creative expression, or experience personal transformation. I recognize the power of art to expand self-understanding, to offer insight not available through other means, and to extend people's ability to communicate. I also view art expressions as personal narratives conveyed through images, as well as through the stories that people attach to those images. Finding personal meaning in one's images is often part of the art therapy process. For some people, it is one of the most potent therapeutic qualities of art expression. It is a powerful way of knowing yourself and a powerful form of healing.

In the coming chapters you will have the chance to see how art therapy works and to experience some of its unique qualities first-hand, through personal art making. But first you will learn where art therapy came from and why it has become important in enhancing health, encouraging emotional transformation, and finding personal meaning.

2

Art Therapy: Drawing on the Past and the Present

Art is the meeting ground of the world inside and the world outside.

ELINOR ULMAN, *ART THERAPY IN THEORY AND PRACTICE*

NOW THAT YOU have some idea about what art therapy is, you may wonder where it came from. Art therapy is a rather new field that has been shaped by many related fields of thought: art, art history, anthropology, psychology, and psychiatry. Its emergence in the twentieth century came about as a result of many unique events. Since art therapy has foundations in both visual art and psychology, there have been many influences, both ancient and modern, which have affected its development and created a growing interest in it since the 1950s.

Art: An Ancient Healer

Art therapy, like many other forms of treatment, has roots that extend far back into history. Since ancient times, art has played a role in health, and symbolic expression has been an important part of healing rituals. The need to make art is a basic human urge, a trait of our species as natural as language, sex, social interaction, and aggression.

Early writing, such as Egyptian hieroglyphics, often used pictures of objects, such as animals and birds. Cuneiform scripts from the Sumerians, logograms of the Mayan culture, and both ancient and contemporary Chinese characters are other examples.

23

Since at least 20,000 B.C., humans have been making marks and images not only to decorate but also to make magic. Stone Age humans were the first image makers; they used primitive implements to sketch figures and forms on cave walls. Because they were preoccupied with protecting themselves from the environment, animals, and unknown forces, they created not only tools and shelters but also images. It is very possible that these early humans tried to ensure a successful hunt by first "capturing" prey through paintings. Some of the most famous of these paintings are found in Europe, deep in caves, which suggests that they were for purposes other than ornamental. Probably they had a magic purpose and were used in rituals rather than merely for decoration.

Humans have consistently created art for purposes of magic, to protect themselves from evil and harm, to express and control powerful emotions such as fear and anxiety, and to prepare themselves for coming events such as hunting. For example, early Egyptians put protective symbols on mummy cases so that mummies would not be destroyed. During the second millennium B.C., the Hittites used different colors of wool in magic rituals for protection. In many cultures, creating and wearing masks was considered to be key to self-preservation and the invocation of special powers. In some African societies, masks were believed to call forth one's ancestors, to ward off dangerous forces, and to help the wearer assume the identity of powerful animals and spirits.

In contemporary cultures as well as preliterate societies, art has been used symbolically to cure illness and bring about both physical and psychological relief. The Navajo, for example, combine song, dance, and sand painting, in which specific patterns are used for specific illnesses. The Tibetans also use sand painting, in the form of a mandala, as a focus for prayer and as an intention for healing and the relief of suffering. The central element in both these examples, the sand painting, is visually symbolic and is intended, in part, for transformation and healing. Humanity's belief that art can be magic, effect change, or transform people and circumstances may be one reason why art has also been viewed as therapeutic.

Shamans are the ancient forerunners of modern psychiatrists and particularly art therapists. The work of the shaman is to bring out harmful and unhealthy elements from people's bodies and to heal mind, body, and spirit using images and rituals. The shaman utilizes visual symbols in his clothing, rituals, and ceremonies to attract spirits, to attain alternate states of consciousness, and to bring about healing. The work of the shaman is strongly connected to the field of art therapy, which uses image making as a modality for health and recovery.

While art may have purposes involving protection, magic, self-preservation, preventive medicine, and physical or psychological healing, the images created by both ancient and contemporary cultures are also intriguing because of their similarities both in meaning and form. There is strong evidence that throughout history humans have had a sense of universal meaning for images and that many visual symbols have recurred over the centuries. Similar marks and configurations have appeared in cultures in different parts of the world, also indicating that there are common meanings for symbols. For example, concentric circles (circles drawn within circles) have been found in Spain, Italy, Australia, Indonesia, Africa, and the Americas. Other shapes and forms, such as spirals, mazelike lines, and circles with perpendicular lines, have repeatedly appeared in the art and design of societies and cultures that had no contact with each other. These occurrences underscore the common bond that humanity has through the visual language of art and its role in the communication of universal concepts.

Art and Mental Illness

Though the ideas that characterize art therapy come partly from ancient and traditional uses of art, they have also been impacted by recent events, particularly the advent of modern psychiatry. In the early twentieth century, psychiatry became increasingly interested in the connections between imagery, human emotion, and the unconscious. This resulted in the belief that art expressions provide tangible evidence as to the nature of a person's inner world. In 1901 Marcel Reja, a French psychiatrist, noted similarities between the art of patients and that of children and primitive artists. As early as 1912, European psychiatrists Emil Kraepelin and Karl Jaspers observed that drawings by patients could be used as aids in understanding psychopathology. However, the door to the relationship between the psyche and visual expression wasn't unlocked until Freud developed his theories of the unconscious and wrote of the images presented in dreams. Freud noted that his patients frequently said they could draw their dreams but were unable to describe them in words. This observation inspired and eventually confirmed the belief that art expression could be a route to understanding the inner world of the human psyche. Freud also included artistic concepts in his clinical work and derived many of his theories from his study of literature and visual art.

Later, Jung formulated the concept of a collective unconscious, with cross-cultural symbols and archetypes that are passed from one generation to the next through art and mythology. Jung had a personal interest in art, and he created drawings, paintings, and carvings throughout his life, recording and exploring his dreams in visual art. Jung realized that all the arts provided ways of accessing feelings and self-understanding; he saw the unconscious mind as a source of well-being and transformation. Jung came to believe that it was important to bring to consciousness emotionally laden images because, if left unconscious, they could have a negative effect on the person's behavior. He felt that dreams, memories, stories, and art could bring forth images hidden in the unconscious.

Jung was particularly interested in the psychological meanings and uses of art expression, especially the mandala, or "magic circle," as well as his own drawings and those of his patients. Unlike Freud, Jung often encouraged patients to draw their dream images. "To paint what we see before us," he said, "is a different art from painting what we see within." Clearly, Jung understood the connection between image and psyche, and he developed a foundation for understanding symbolic meanings in imagery through his studies of archetypes and universalities inherent in visual art.

Both Freud's and Jung's explanations of images in art and dreams attracted the psychiatric community and generated interest in artistic expression within the psychoanalytic profession. Their interpretations of the unconscious processes of the mind also provided psychiatry with a basis for using art expressions and dreams in psychoanalysis. Through Freud's and Jung's writings, psychotherapists began to realize that language was not always adequate and that images, either in the form of art or dreams, could provide information that words alone could not. The idea that expression through images was symbolic began to take hold, and there was increasing attention to understanding and finding meaning for patients' images as sources of unconscious or repressed thoughts and emotions.

Around the turn of the century, interest also arose in the artwork of people with mental illness. In 1872 Ambroise Tardieu, a highly respected French psychiatrist, published a book on mental illness that included a brief outline of what he thought were the characteristics of artwork created by people determined to be insane. In 1876 and 1888 Paul-Max Simon, a French psychiatrist, published a more comprehensive series of studies of the drawings of people with mental illness. Simon has been referred to as the "father of art and psychiatry" and was one of the first psychiatrists to establish a large collection of drawings and paintings by patients in insane asylums. He has been credited with influencing the diagnostic uses of drawings, based on his belief that symptoms could be related to the content of artwork.

During the 1920s Hans Prinzhorn, an art historian turned psychiatrist, began soliciting patients' drawings, paintings, and sculptures from other doctors and hospitals throughout Germany, Switzerland, Italy, Austria, and the Netherlands. He collected five thousand pieces by more than five hundred patients, works that would later become the basis of his publication *Artistry of the Mentally Ill* and the contemporary phenomenon known as outsider art (Figure 2.1). Instead of studying the psychopathology of the artists in his collection, Prinzhorn was more interested in their creative process and the visual forms they created. He believed that humankind's fundamental drive was toward self-expression and communication and that it included the urge to play, decorate, symbolize, and organize ideas into visual forms. Prinzhorn held that the creative process of art making is basic to all people, with or without mental illness, and that art was a natural way to achieve psychological integration and wellness. He maintained that art making was "a universal creative urge" and that even those afflicted with illness could express themselves through art.

Prinzhorn's ideas were compatible with Jung's ideas about archetypes and the collective unconscious. While he accepted the notion of an unconscious mind, he rejected the idea that art could be

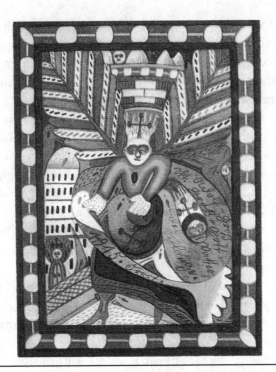

Figure 2.1 Painting from the Prinzhorn Collection, date unknown
(Reprinted from Artistry of the Mentally Ill *© 1972 by Hans Prinzhorn, with permission of Springer-Velag KG)*

reduced to clinical analysis. He saw art as a method of self-discovery for individuals with mental illness and perhaps even an avenue to mental wellness.

At about the same time Prinzhorn was beginning to collect the art of people with mental illness, Walter Morgenthaler, a Swiss psychiatrist, published a book on the art of Adolph Wolfli, who suffered from schizophrenia. Wolfli was confined to a psychiatric hospital for more than thirty years, and while there, he made numerous drawings that are known for their detail, complexity, and color (Figure 2.2). Like the artists in the Prinzhorn Collection, Wolfli had no formal art training and worked spontaneously with what limited materials he had.

Interest in the psychopathology of artistic expression has continued into recent times. Art historians, psychiatrists, mental health

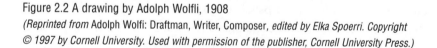

Figure 2.2 A drawing by Adolph Wolfli, 1908
(Reprinted from Adolph Wolfi: Draftman, Writer, Composer, *edited by Elka Spoerri. Copyright © 1997 by Cornell University. Used with permission of the publisher, Cornell University Press.)*

professionals, art therapists, and artists have an ongoing fascination with the art of people with mental illness. For the most part, these individuals have had no formal training and create spontaneous works with unique styles and content. Their art is often visually beautiful, and some artists and art historians have valued its naive or primitive qualities.

Art and Diagnosis

Interest in the meaning of art created by people with mental illness led to increased interest in using images and drawing to diagnose and evaluate mental conditions. The concept of projective testing emerged in an attempt to develop standard tasks so that comparisons could be made between normal behavior and abnormal responses. The term *projection* refers to the tendency to attribute to others feelings or perceptions that one experiences. Leonardo da Vinci was thought to have inadvertently created one of the first projective tests when he observed his own associations to a paint blot made by throwing a sponge against a wall. "Various experiences can be seen in such a blot," he wrote, "provided one wants to find them in it—human heads, various animals, battle, cliffs, seas, clouds, or forests and other things."

The Rorschach test, which was first published in Europe in the early 1920s and shortly after in the United States, is a series of inkblots designed to evoke associations and emotions from the viewer. It was named after its creator, Hermann Rorschach, who believed that there was a relationship between an individual's personality and how he or she perceived shapes and colors. In the Rorschach test, ten inkblots with different colors, forms, and configurations are shown—one at a time and in a definite order—to a person. The person is asked to describe what he or she sees in each card. The test was originally used as a form of free association that could be interpreted by a psychologist or psychiatrist. While today the Rorschach test is not considered to be a reliable test of personality, it was part of the early trend toward seeing art expressions and images as ways to help understand and decipher the unconscious mind.

Drawings also began to be studied for possible indications of mental illness. In 1906 Fritz Mohr, a German psychiatrist, described the first drawing tests for psychological purposes. In 1926 Florence Goodenough developed a drawing test for children designed to measure intelligence through the number of details in their drawings of a man. Goodenough and other researchers at that time realized that this Draw-a-Man test might reveal not only intelligence but also personality characteristics. Other tests were developed in the 1940s to assess personality through drawing. Since that time, both children's and adults' drawings have been considered to be representations of emotional and internal states, although research to support this idea is inconsistent. Nonetheless, interest in how drawings may project personality continues today.

Artists and Psychology

While artists have always searched for meaning in their imagery and have explored the power of creativity to heal and cope, the advent of psychiatry and psychology in the early twentieth century had a powerful impact on many artists' work. Freud's concept of the unconscious became important. The unconscious is defined as the part of the mind not available to consciousness; it is displayed in behavior such as slips of the tongue, dissociated actions, and dreams.

Surrealism is a twentieth-century style that was influenced by Freudian psychology; it was based on the idea that imagery came from the unconscious. Surrealists were also interested in dream imagery. They believed that dreams contained meanings that could be interpreted, a concept that Freud proposed. Artists such as Salvador Dalí and Max Ernst included symbolic images in their works. The surrealists sought to create art that contained fantastic or shocking content similar to the images experienced in dreams. They emphasized the need to go beyond reproducing external reality and to bring to light the inner world of the individual.

Techniques such as automatic drawing interested artists like Joan Miró. These artists believed that through spontaneous or automatic drawing, they could reach and express the unconscious mind. Later, artist Jackson Pollock (who was undergoing psychoanalysis at the time of his famous "drip" paintings) used a painting method called psychic automatism to help express his inner thoughts and ideas on canvas. This method involved generating images from the unconscious mind and painting in an unrestrained manner. Pollock, like many of his contemporaries, was convinced that the unconscious played a major role in his art.

Expressionism, an art movement that emphasized the depiction of emotion, also underscored the exploration of the artist's inner world. Most of Paul Gauguin's and Vincent van Gogh's work is clearly expressionistic, because of their emotionally laden use of color and brushstrokes. In the early twentieth century, Wassily Kandinsky and other painters used abstract forms and pure colors to communicate feelings and evoke an emotional response from the viewer. Kandinsky, in particular, explored both psychological and spiritual concerns through dramatic and spontaneous use of color, lines, and shapes. He believed that his work reflected the free flow of unconscious thought.

For Kandinsky, other expressionists, and surrealist painters, art was rendered with a spontaneity like that of the psychological process of free association. At the same time, free association (the process of allowing one's consciousness to flow from thought to thought, without intention or censorship) was being explored by Freud as a method of clinically understanding the unconscious mind and human behavior. While psychiatry was attempting to understand the inner workings of the mind, artists also began to look inward for images for their work.

Other artists explored the spontaneity of "nonartists," such as children and people with mental illness. Jean Dubuffet is one of many artists who have worked in the style of art brut, or "art in the raw." Dubuffet was influenced by artwork in the Prinzhorn and Morgenthaler collections and began to create art based on the art of children and people with mental illness. While Prinzhorn and Morgenthaler saw the works of people with mental illness as examples of humankind's instinct to create, Dubuffet regarded the work as unique and original art, valuing its spontaneity.

This fascination with the unique and talented work of the untrained artist continues today, and artists, art historians, and critics have come to value what is now known as outsider art. Outsider art is an important concept, because it recognizes that artistic creativity is a shared human experience that transcends disability or environment. This recognition helped set the stage for further exploration into the artistic expressions of people who have a psychiatric disability and those who are marginalized by society, such as prisoners, the physically disabled, and the elderly.

Artists, Creativity, and Madness

If you have taken an art history course or read biographies of artists, you may have wondered why many creative people seem to have led emotionally tortured or psychologically complicated lives. There has been some question about the connections between creativity and madness. Plato noted that artists were endowed by the gods with a "divine madness," connoting a more positive view of creativity as a personal quality and as a talent or gift. Others have viewed the relationship between the creative process of art making and the relationship between visual art and mental health in a different light.

It is true that many of the greatest artists, composers, and writers have suffered from mental illness. In her book *Touched with Fire*, researcher Kay Redfield Jamison observes this to be true, according to psychiatry's current diagnostic criteria. Manic-depressive illness can cause dramatic, cyclical shifts in energy levels, mood, behavior, and thought patterns. Depression causes melancholy, low energy, apathy, hopelessness, and, in some cases, thoughts of suicide. According to Jamison, recent studies indicate that a high percentage of artists—visual artists, writers, poets, and composers—meet the diagnostic criteria for manic-depressive illness or major depression. She notes that these mental illnesses can sometimes enhance or possibly contribute to creative abilities in some people.

One of the better-known cases of an artist who probably suffered from a mood disorder is that of Vincent van Gogh. Van Gogh's family also suffered with depression and manic-depressive illness. His brother Theo was depressed, his youngest brother, Cornelius, was reported to have committed suicide, and his sister, Wilhelmina, had a psychotic illness, possibly schizophrenia.

Biographers report that Vincent as a child was depressed, a quality that continued into his adulthood. He believed, however, that his sadness and inner turmoil fueled his creativity as a painter. There were manic aspects to van Gogh as well. During the eight years of his career as an artist, he created approximately eight hundred works, four hundred of them in the last year of his life.

While it seems that van Gogh was manic-depressive, more than one hundred diagnoses have been offered, including schizophrenia, brain tumor, epilepsy, syphilis, and absinthe poisoning, an addiction that may have contributed to his manic-depressive disorder. Van Gogh reported that he heard voices, had blackouts during which he lost consciousness, behaved aggressively at times, and felt disoriented. He tried suicide on several occasions by swallowing toxic paints and turpentine.

For many years there has been speculation about the style and images in the paintings of van Gogh and their connection to his behavior and depression. It is obvious from what we know about van Gogh through historical accounts and his own writings that he was emotionally tormented. Art historians and psychiatrists have pointed to van Gogh's swirling brushstrokes as indicative of his manic episodes. The artist himself noted in a letter written during the last summer of his life, "I am painting immense expanses of wheat beneath troubled skies, and I have not hesitated to express sadness, extreme solitude." Van Gogh's final painting, *Wheat Field with Crows* (Figure 2.3), depicts a scene with a dark sky, stormy weather, and a large flock of black crows, often referred to as possible omens of his troubled emotional state and pending suicide.

Cases like van Gogh's and others have intrigued people interested in the connections between art and illness and raised questions about how art expressions reflect psychological problems or emotional distress. Some speculate that psychological problems and emotional distress compel some people to make art. Certainly, some of what is considered the world's greatest art, such as van Gogh's work, comes from emotional suffering. Many artists consider misfortunes to be the inspiration and drive for their art making.

But creativity is not always the result of emotional turmoil. In *The Courage to Create*, psychologist Rollo May notes, "The creative process must be explored not as a product of sickness but as representing the highest degree of emotional health, as the expression of normal people in the act of actualizing themselves." May

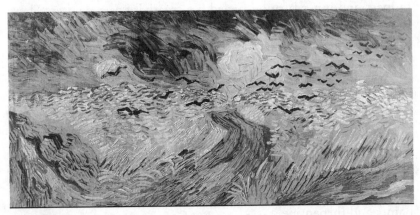

Figure 2.3 *Wheat Field with Crows*, by Vincent van Gogh
(Reprinted with permission of the Van Gogh Museum and the Vincent van Gogh Foundation, Amsterdam)

also observes that creative people may be special in that they can live with emotional distress and have the ability to transform it into creative works.

Does mental illness cause people to become more creative? While evidence of this connection is inconclusive, artists with mood disorders such as depression often report that their condition is a source not only of turmoil but also of inspiration and creative thinking. It is true that creativity has helped some people transform conflicts, relieve emotional distress, and explore personal crisis, pain, and psychological turmoil.

While some scholars have related creativity and artistic genius to madness and emotional disorders, many people have found art to be their salvation from mental illness and traumatic experiences. Creativity for them is a means of coping with anxiety, depression, and disturbing emotions, rather than the result of psychological problems.

Art Therapy: An Idea Whose Time Had Arrived

The twentieth century brought with it the advent of psychoanalysis, artists' interest in symbolic and spontaneous images, psychiatry's interest in the art of the mentally ill, and the development of projective testing. Like most therapies of the time, art therapy grew from the psychoanalytic movement and beliefs about the symbolic content of images that could be derived from patients' art expressions and dreams. By midcentury there was also a growing belief that the creative process of art making could encourage rehabilitation, change, and growth. Both a growing interest in images as representations of the unconscious and the therapeutic potential of the creative process helped open the door for the emergence of the field of art therapy.

There were other important events that paved the way for art therapy. The development of new therapies and treatment approaches dramatically increased after 1950, creating an atmosphere that encouraged the appearance and acceptance of novel methods of treatment. Some of these therapeutic approaches originated in the nineteenth century in the United States and Europe, when a more humane treatment of mental patients, called moral therapy, was initiated. Moral therapy included sending patients to country retreats where they received personal attention in the form of occupational training and the arts, including painting. The movement lasted only a few years, but it resurfaced in the twentieth century in what were eventually known as milieu therapies. Increasingly, hospitals, clinics, and rehabilitation centers began to include not only visual art but also music, movement, and creative writing along with "talk therapies." The arts began to be used in tandem with traditional treatment to help clients work through, identify, and understand feelings, thoughts, perceptions, and experiences.

Consequently, the art therapies (not only art, but also music, dance/movement, drama, and poetry) became fields of study in their own right and were increasingly recognized as viable treatment options for hospitalized individuals. The field of art therapy emerged and gained attention in health care facilities throughout the United States and within psychiatry, psychology, education, and the arts. Although many individuals were involved in the beginnings of art therapy and many had discovered the healing power of art, two people are thought to be primarily responsible for art therapy in the United States.

The introduction of art as a therapeutic modality is attributed to Margaret Naumburg in the 1940s. Naumburg is considered to be one of the first to delineate art therapy as a distinctive form of psychotherapy. She viewed art expression as a way to manifest unconscious imagery, an observation resonant with the predominant psychoanalytic viewpoint of the early twentieth century. However, she took Freud's concepts one step further by having her clients draw their dreams and images rather than only talk about them. In Naumburg's view the primary value of art therapy was in authentic expression and in communication; she considered the images produced by clients to be a form of symbolic speech.

In the 1950s art therapist Edith Kramer proposed that the healing potential of art making stemmed from the ability of creative work to activate certain psychological processes. Kramer stressed creativity, not merely communication of visually symbolic speech, as key to the art therapy process. She observed that the act of creating an artistic product involves channeling, reduction, and transformation of inner experiences and can be an act of sublimation, integration, and synthesis. Although art expression cannot directly resolve conflict, it can provide a place where new attitudes and feelings can be expressed and tried out. Thus Kramer's view of art therapy is more deeply embedded in the art process than Naumburg's product-oriented philosophy.

Others had a major influence on the early development of art therapy. Hanna Yaxa Kwiatkowska, an art therapist who worked at the National Institute of Mental Health in the 1950s and 1960s, introduced art therapy into family therapy sessions. She believed that specific drawing activities were helpful in identifying family members' roles and status and in providing a therapeutic experience of working together. Later, in the 1960s and 1970s, art therapist Janie Rhyne used art expression to help people achieve self-awareness and self-actualization (that is, the attainment of one's fullest potential and a sense of satisfaction with one's life). Rhyne emphasized the person's own interpretation of art expressions and the person-centered approach to therapy popular during that time. Thanks to such advocates, art therapy had become a recognized field by the 1960s.

At about the same time the field of art therapy was emerging in the United States, it was also being discovered and developed in Europe. Artist Adrian Hill discovered the value of art making during his stay at a sanatorium in England as a tuberculosis patient in the 1940s. He began to develop the idea of art therapy as treatment for physical and emotional illness, and, by Hill's own account, he was the first art therapist. Like others in the United States at this time, Hill believed that art making alleviated the monotony of hospitalization and provided a sense of hope for a person facing serious illness. Hill's ideas became an important basis for art therapy in medical settings.

Edward Adamson, another early art therapist in England, worked as an artist with patients in a hospital studio. In 1946 Adamson provided patients with an environment in which to paint and "to cure themselves." He realized that art making was a unique way for individuals to contribute to their own treatment. Rather than analyzing the art expressions of patients, as others of this time did, he believed that the artistic expressions spoke for themselves and were a testimony to the healing qualities of the art process. Adamson compiled a collection of sixty thousand paintings and objects by people with mental illness, which now constitute the Adamson Collection in England.

While many individuals contributed to the emergence and early development of art therapy as a distinct field, one hospital was particularly influential: the Menninger Clinic, in Topeka, Kansas. The Menninger Clinic, a world-famous psychiatric facility, was founded by Charles Menninger and his two sons, Karl and William, in 1925. As psychiatrists, the Menningers felt that art could help patients recover from mental illness, and they encouraged the development of activity therapies. In the 1930s they introduced art therapy to their facility when they invited artist Mary Huntoon to offer art classes to psychiatric patients. Huntoon, who was trained as an artist, not as a psychologist, helped patients use art to process and release emotional problems and trauma. She coined the word *art-synthesis* to describe the process of self-discovery that many of her patients experienced after completing an artwork. She felt that the therapeutic value of art was in the making of it, rather than in analyzing it for diagnostic or symbolic meaning. Through creating a drawing, a painting, or another artwork, patients had the opportunity to experience catharsis and discover their own meaning for their art expressions.

The Menninger Clinic continued to have a major influence on the development of art therapy in the United States throughout the decades that followed. Other artists worked at the Menninger during the 1950s and 1960s. Two of them, Don Jones and Robert Ault, were instrumental in forming (in 1969) the American Art Therapy Association, a national organization of art therapists, making art therapy a recognized professional field.

Mind, Body, and Spirit

Several other important influences on the development of art therapy are worth mentioning. The first is the impact of alternative or complementary medicine on the field of health care in recent years.

Alternative or complementary medicine refers to medical practices that usually involve natural or holistic means to promote wellness. It has been reported that one-third of all Americans and that 70 percent of people fifty years of age or older use some form of alternative or complementary treatment, either to maintain health or to supplement medical treatment they are already receiving.

The phrase *mind-body intervention* is often used when referring to alternative and/or complementary approaches to treatment. Since the 1970s, there has been a growing movement to explore the mind's capacity to influence the body. Practitioners in the fields of medicine and psychology began to realize that the mind-body connection was important to treatment and that therapies could have a simultaneous impact on mind and body. The placebo—a procedure that has no intrinsic therapeutic value and yet provides positive results—is one of the most widely recognized examples of mind-body interactions.

Many of the newer alternative treatments are based on the belief that the mind and body are connected. Most of today's mind-body procedures and philosophies, including art therapy, are not new but are founded on earlier concepts and practices. The need to acknowledge the patient's mind in relation to illness has been recognized since the time of Hippocrates. Until the nineteenth century, those who wrote about medicine and healing practices often noted the influence of negative emotions on the onset and course of illness, as well as positive emotions such as hope, faith, peacefulness, and confidence.

Well-known mind-body interventions include meditation, mental imagery, hypnosis, biofeedback, prayer, and support groups. Psychotherapy is also considered a mind-body intervention in that it addresses a person's emotional and mental health, which is connected to physical health. Any of these therapies may help people experience and express their illness in new ways. They may also help people come to a feeling of being healed rather than cured, meaning that the person has reached a sense of psychological or spiritual well-being even though his or her illness is still present.

Spiritual practices have also been recognized by the medical establishment for its therapeutic potential. Spiritual practices are not necessarily beliefs or values found in formal religions, but to one's inner sense of something greater than oneself and to one's ability to find meaning that transcends life's problems. Prayer, religious attendance, and spiritual belief systems have been found to be important factors in health and well-being and, in some cases, in remission or recovery from trauma or serious illness.

Art making has also been widely recognized for its deep connection to mind, body, and spirit. Through art making a person can explore, express, and confront issues that relate to all three of these areas. Emotional conflicts may be addressed, physical symptoms may be faced and accepted, and spiritual experiences such as hope and transcendence may be realized through the creative process. As a result, art therapy has been acknowledged as a "mind-body intervention" by the National Center for Complementary and Alternative Medicine, in recognition of the power of self-expression and the creative process in mental, physical, and spiritual health.

Creativity in Counseling and Psychotherapy

Art therapists often use verbal counseling in their work with people, combining traditional talk therapy along with art making. Not surprisingly, mental health counselors, social workers, marriage and family counselors, and psychologists have also used various forms of visual arts and other modalities to facilitate their clients' exploration of thoughts and feelings. Counseling educator Samuel Gladding notes that counseling at its best capitalizes on creativity to help individuals to express themselves personally and uniquely. From this belief, the creativity in counseling movement emerged, embracing the idea that all the creative arts invigorate and enliven verbal counseling and traditional talk therapy. Counseling—which includes art, music, movement, and other forms of expression—encourages playfulness, divergent thinking, flexibility, humor, risk taking, independence, and openness. These qualities are believed to be strongly associated with personal creativity and a healthy personality.

Like art therapists, creative counselors and psychotherapists believe that increasing an individual's capacity for creative thinking and behavior through drawing, painting, constructing, or using one's imagination helps to reduce emotional distress and conflict and enhances understanding of oneself and others. Ultimately, these creative behaviors may contribute to good mental health, helping people of all ages become more adaptive, resilient, and productive when confronted with life's stresses.

Arts in Health Care

In the past two decades, there has been a growing interest in bringing the visual arts and other modalities, such as dance, music, drama, creative writing, and humor, into health care settings. Out of this interest, the arts in health care movement developed, recognizing the special power of the arts to promote wellness through self-expression and creativity.

Examples of this application of arts in health care include bringing the visual arts into medical settings, such as hospitals and rehabilitation centers, with the help of art therapists, artists in residence, arts coordinators, activity therapists, physicians, and other health care professionals; setting up patient art exhibits or bringing in artwork to enrich hospital environments; and decorating hospital interiors, such as waiting rooms and offices, to enhance and humanize the space. The function of arts medicine is similar to the goal of art therapy—to use art as part of the recovery and healing process.

Recently, visual artists have also become interested in the arts in health care settings to promote health and wellness in patients of all ages. While not formally trained in psychology or medicine, these artists seek to understand how art making can facilitate well-being in a variety of ways. Some may create art or aesthetically pleasing environments that are intended to heal the viewers. They might use symbolic images that are designed to calm and center, activate a physiological response, or induce a transcendent experience. For example, a painter may create images intended to heal and balance the viewer through the use of specific lighting, color, and imagery. Many artists have used the creative process to explore its healing for themselves or to make art that expresses their experiences with illness, pain, and the process of healing. Darcy Lynn, whose work is described in Chapter 8, has used painting to help in her recovery from lymphoma and to record her experiences with life-threatening illness.

Art therapists and artists may bring art activities to the bedsides of patients with cancer, physical injuries, or other medical conditions. They may also design art programs to enhance medical treatments, reduce pain, and induce relaxation. Both art therapists and artists who use art in health care agree that the creative process of art making is life affirming and can stimulate possibilities for growth, transformation, and self-understanding.

Community Arts

Artists, because of their direct experience with the process of art making, have long understood the potential of art to express and make sense of our inner world. Some have recognized that this potential can be harnessed to bring positive changes to neighborhoods, inner cities, and communities.

In *The Re-enchantment of Art*, Suzi Gablik notes that artists are becoming interested in making art that is socially responsible, transformative, and healing. She refers to this phenomenon as "making art as if the world mattered," an approach that emphasizes connection and empathy rather than creating art for art's sake. Some artists who embrace this idea have chosen to collaborate with populations that society may have written off as unreachable. Raw Art Works (RAW), in Lynn, Massachusetts, provides visual arts to at-risk children and adolescents who are marginalized by society because of ethnicity or low income. It offers hands-on arts programs in schools, neighborhoods, soup kitchens, housing developments, detention centers, and its own studios, inviting youth to examine their lives and their roles in their communities (Figure 2.4). Participants in RAW's programs are given the opportunity to be creative, to participate in meaningful collaborations with others, and to achieve a sense of self-worth and personal identity.

For more than twenty years, the Art Studio, part of the Center for Therapy Through the Arts in Cleveland, Ohio, offers unique, innovative community-based art therapy programs. Community-based studios provide places where individuals with special needs and older adults participate in creative arts classes. Programs also serve autistic and behaviorally challenged children, individuals with

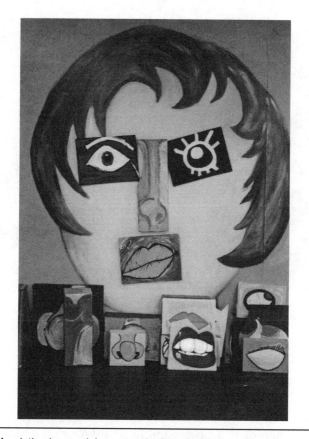

Figure 2.4 A painting by an adolescent at the Raw Art Works program
(Reprinted with permission of RAW Arts)

brain or spinal cord injuries, and adults with Alzheimer's disease, developmentally disadvantaged people, and those suffering from depression or other emotional disorders. WheelArt—Rolling Toward Wellness is part of the innovative treatment of patients confined to wheelchairs due to spinal cord injuries. Rolling through brightly colored pools of paint with wheelchairs, physically challenged artists create vibrant patterns of color and patterns on T-shirts, socks, aprons, and other items (Figure 2.5). Many individuals who are otherwise unable to find a creative means of expression participate in this integrated effort where their contributions are unique and esteemed.

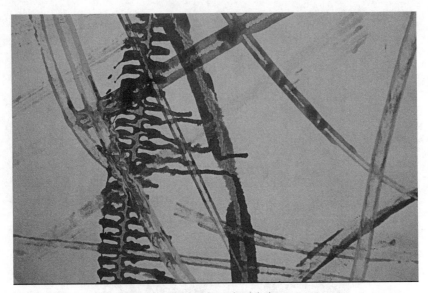

Figure 2.5 A WheelArt painting created with a wheelchair
(Reprinted with permission of the Center for Therapy Through the Arts)

Art Therapy Today

Today, art therapy is a profession in its own right, and guidelines for practice and training have been established. Because the arts are interrelated, art therapy did not come about in isolation. Other disciplines that recognize the unique role of art in therapy have developed simultaneously. The expressive therapies, expressive arts therapies, or creative arts therapies (art, music, drama, movement, and poetry) also have become important treatment methods. Expressive therapists or expressive arts therapists utilize all arts modalities in their work, a practice referred to as intermodal expressive therapy. Intermodal techniques are based on the idea that all arts have qualities in common and can be integrated and used in therapy.

While some art therapists are also expressive therapists by training or credentials, art therapists are generally considered part of the larger group of practitioners, creative arts therapists. Just as there are art therapists, there are music therapists, dance/movement therapists, poetry therapists, and drama therapists. Each of these creative arts therapies has its own unique theoretical foundation, training, and applications.

Visual art has been celebrated not only for its aesthetic and decorative value and as a record of historical events but also for its potential to help us express and understand ourselves. The emergence of art therapy at this time in history is not surprising, given the increased interest in art as a means of communication and in such areas as the psychological meanings of visual symbols, the relationship between creativity and health, and alternative methods of treatment and healing. In a sense, it seems that humankind has come full circle in its realization that art making is an important means of expressing mind, body, and soul and that it is intimately connected to health and well-being.

In the next two chapters you will learn more about how you can benefit from art making and why art therapy is personally enriching, life enhancing, and transformative.

3

Getting Started:
Drawing from Within

Art is a way of knowing what we actually believe.

PAT B. ALLEN, *ART IS A WAY OF KNOWING*

IN ANY FORM of therapy or personal growth experience, it is important to set the stage. In art therapy this may involve learning a new way of experiencing art and discovering how you express yourself through visual images. It also may include learning how to use your intuition, rediscovering your sense of play and exploration, and making time in your life for art making.

When I work with children, they are generally excited to make art. For them, it is a natural means of communicating and interacting. Most adults who come to my practice or workshops, however, have not made art for many years, in many cases not since they were very young children. Others have tried art as therapy on their own but need some guidance in how to develop and deepen their experiences with art. Since everyone's experience of art is unique, it is important to consider how each individual's experience may influence his or her perception of art making when beginning to use art as therapy. As an art therapist, I am concerned with helping people feel comfortable with art making, whether by discovering their visual language through various materials or by recognizing how their beliefs may prevent them from enjoying the art-making process.

As I said earlier, understanding art therapy is difficult unless you experience it for yourself. For this reason, I have included some art therapy activities throughout the book. These are very basic art experientials, similar to those that art therapists might use. Each experiential is designed both to help you learn more about art therapy and to introduce you to the value of personal art making. These activities require simple materials and supplies that are discussed in detail in Chapter 5.

These activities are not intended to be a substitute for art therapy. They are designed to provide a starting place for using art as therapy, to familiarize you with the concept of images as reflections of your inner world, and to demonstrate how art making can be therapeutic. As an art therapist, I believe that art making has the potential to enhance everyone's health and well-being, and one purpose of this book is to help you discover its potential in your life. While the field of art therapy has, for the most part, focused on using art in the treatment of mental illness, emotional distress, and disability, art therapy is also a useful approach with healthy people or, as I like to say, "normal neurotics" like you and me. Art therapy is not confined to the treatment of people with mental or physical illness. Rather, it is a useful and powerful method of self-understanding and expression for all people. As noted in the first two chapters of this book, it is a fundamental extension of our need to create, experiment, express, and make special. For this reason, art making has the potential to increase your internal sense of health and well-being.

However, to get the most from this book and to fully explore the exercises, it also may be helpful to experience them with a therapist's guidance and feedback or as part of a group or in an art studio where your experience can be more fully supported. An art therapist or another therapist with training in art therapy can help deepen your experience and will assist you with any questions or concerns you have along the way. Support groups can be particularly helpful because they generally have a leader, therapist, or facilitator to assist you, as well as group members who are available to listen and reflect your feelings and experiences. You may also want to try an art therapy group or an art studio geared to helping people make art for the purpose of self-exploration and insight; some of these types of groups are discussed in Chapter 9.

Many individuals have discovered, either serendipitously or through the advice and encouragement of a family member or friend, that art making is a form of personal therapy for them. Some have read or heard of other people who used art as a healing element in their lives, whether to overcome trauma, confront loss, or recover from illness. While some individuals have found healing, transformation, and insight through exploring and making art on their own, many of us need to have the help and guidance of a professional in exploring ourselves through art. Chapter 10 describes ways of continuing and deepening your exploration, and the resources section at the end of the book provides additional information on where to find a therapist or group to further your experience of art therapy.

Nonartists and Art Therapy

Some people who come to art therapy have already had significant experiences with art making, perhaps through taking art classes, reading popular drawing books, or studying painting through books or tapes. I often receive calls from people who already paint, sculpt, or take photographs and want to explore art therapy for personal growth or to work on specific issues through their art with the help of an art therapist. Some, having studied art in college or at a formal art school, consider themselves to be artists. People who consider themselves to be visual artists may already see their art making as a form of therapy. The artists with whom I work often bring samples of their work with them to art therapy sessions and usually feel very comfortable with art as a form of self-expression.

You may wonder if being an artist makes art therapy easier, because an artist is already familiar with using art for self-expression. You may be surprised that the vast majority of people I work with in art therapy have not had many art experiences and consider themselves to be nonartists. Having artistic training does not always make art therapy easier. In fact, some people with artistic talent find the process of art therapy a little difficult. Art therapy asks you to experience art making in a somewhat different way from traditional art classes.

Before becoming an art therapist, I had several years of training as a professional artist and designer. My training in fine arts and design taught me many things important to success in creating art for exhibition and sale, including use of color, composition, and technique. I learned how to paint in a traditional way by copying masterpieces in a museum, and I worked at making meticulous copies of the human skeleton in order to achieve the skills necessary to make "fine art." Through formal art training I learned the academics of painting, drawing, sculpture, and design, information that helped me feel successful as a visual artist and designer.

Using art for therapy, personal exploration, self-understanding, and insight took my art making in a very different direction. Art therapy asked me to create art from an inner world. It also proposed that all art is acceptable, that there are no rules about how to paint or draw, and that there is no right or wrong way to make art. When as a trained artist I was first confronted with the idea of art therapy, I struggled to put aside some of the rules I had established. As a designer, I had learned successful ways of developing patterns and images, often very tight and controlled graphics. My work as a painter also involved specific training in the use of color and the creation of contemporary abstract works on large canvases, a trend in the art world at that time. Making art as a means of self-exploration and personal growth was a new experience for me, and it forced me to look at how I defined art, art making, and creativity.

While the idea of art therapy intrigued me, it initially was difficult to let go of some of the beliefs I had accumulated through years of studio art training. Although I was appreciative of my art training, I was also excited to have found a field that valued other purposes for art making. The focus on the importance of "drawing from within" and the emphasis on the process of self-exploration rather than creating a technically perfect product provided a refreshing and meaningful direction for both my art and my own journey of self-discovery.

Many nonartists find art therapy easier to understand than do some visual artists. If you have not had many experiences with art making, you probably have fewer preconceptions to overcome. You probably haven't developed an artistic style (such as my early focus on design and the technical aspects of painting) that may interfere with the art therapy process. In any case, you still have unique impressions about art, art making, and creativity. We all have notions about what art is and what it is supposed to look like. When we're given the opportunity to make art, these notions influence our response.

Experiencing the art activities in this book, especially if you consider yourself to be a nonartist, is like beginning a new language.

Art expression is a form of nonverbal communication, and, like any language, it takes time to learn how to communicate through it. Depending on your experiences with art, the process of art therapy may seem foreign to you at first and even uncomfortable. As an adult, you may not have had any exposure to art making for many years, and you may feel out of touch with your creative self. When you start to experience art as a form of therapy, it is important to think about these personal experiences with art making.

Your Personal Art History

When adults who come to my practice or workshops identify themselves as nonartists, it generally means that they have not tried drawing or painting since childhood, and their last experiences were elementary-school art classes as young children. In preschool or elementary school, art is an important form of communication for most of us. You may remember coloring, cutting, and pasting colored paper as a young child; you may have looked forward to art class each week or worked with an art teacher who came to visit your school on occasion. By the time children are ten or eleven, however, art often takes a backseat to reading, writing, mathematics, and other activities. Drawing, painting, and making things with one's hands and imagination become less important than other ways of communicating and are replaced with different activities during preadolescence and adolescence. As a result, most of us lose touch with what was once a natural activity of childhood. As an adult, you may feel that you cannot make art or draw or that you do not have any talent.

Also, as preteenagers, many people become discouraged with art making and may not draw or paint again, except if they are encouraged by parents or take art courses in middle or high school. During this age children become very interested in making drawings look real, but they are usually not skilled in creating the three-dimensional perspective necessary to achieve photographically realistic images. This frustration, along with the other influences previously mentioned, causes most children to give up art in favor of other activities and ways of expressing themselves. People continue to progress in other areas of development, such as language, but the development of art-making skills may not persist. For this reason, many drawings done by adults without any more recent art-making experiences (including those of you reading this book) look like children's drawings at the age of ten or eleven.

More personal influences may have stopped you from making art. You may remember an event or a time when you decided that you were not an artist, were not creative, or did not have artistic talent. I have heard countless stories from clients, colleagues, and people who attend my training workshops, recalling the exact moment when they decided that they had no artistic talent. Sometimes people remember a particular person who ridiculed their art, misunderstood what they were trying to communicate, or gave them a poor grade in an art class.

In the art therapy training workshops that I conduct with counselors and psychologists, people often get anxious when I tell them that we are going to make some art. People who come for art therapy as patients or clients can have a similar feeling of dread. They may wonder how to begin or if they can really benefit from art making in some way. Some people even apologize before they get started, thinking that they are not skilled or talented enough to participate. These reactions usually come from our childhood or adolescence, when a teacher, a family member, or another authority figure criticized a drawing, a painting, or an object we made. Art books, art history courses, and television documentaries on "great" artists can also cause us to think that art is an activity only for the very talented or those with special skills.

When people hear that I am an art therapist, they often spontaneously relate a memory of childhood art making, often a traumatic one that caused them to be fearful of art making as adults. Most people do not realize that how they see art making as adults has a great deal to do with their experiences as children. We carry memories of these experiences with us throughout our lives. Luckily, most of us have had some positive experiences. Some of us remember a paint-by-number set, a piece of needlework, or an art project in school that earned an A. Unfortunately, the negative experiences may be easier to remember. Some of these memories may prevent us from engaging in art making or other creative endeavors as adults, fearing that we will fail or that we are not truly artists.

Over many years of work with adults, I have often heard them relate painful memories of being unable to draw or feeling uncomfortable about expressing themselves through art. They also may relate frustration with the process of drawing (for example, "I can't make it look real" or "I am not talented in art"), just as children in this stage speak of their frustration with perfecting the realism of their drawings. Others may remember someone's uncomplimentary remarks about the drawings they made as children, perhaps a thoughtless comment from a teacher, family member, or friend. My friend and colleague Ewa, who holds a doctoral degree in anthropology and two master's degrees, told me that she clearly remembers her elementary-school teacher proclaiming, "What a nice sewing machine!" upon looking at her drawing of a horse. Obviously, she was discouraged by the teacher's comments. It was a particularly impressionable time in her drawing development, and Ewa observes that she never felt comfortable with art again.

Ewa's story reminds me of Antoine de St. Exupéry's tale *The Little Prince*. In the first chapter, the author tells how he once drew a picture of a snake that had swallowed an elephant. To his dismay, the adults who looked at his picture said it looked like a hat. When he tried to show them that this was indeed a drawing of a snake with an elephant inside it, they continued to discount his description, misunderstanding the meaning of his picture. Sadly, he related that he never wanted to draw again after that experience. I think the incident that St. Exupéry describes is common and often unfortunately causes both children and adults to put down their pencils and brushes, never to draw, paint, or create again.

Because people may have stopped expressing themselves through art for many different reasons, I often explore childhood memories of art making with the people I see in my practice and in workshops. Some of your childhood memories may recall negative messages you received about art, but you may also recall many positive experiences. Perhaps you remember a supportive parent, grandparent, or teacher who encouraged and nurtured your creative talents or recall a time when you made a special drawing or an object that gave you pride and satisfaction.

Before beginning any of the experientials in this book, remember that early negative experiences with art making can prevent you

Your Personal Art History

- What was art in your life, growing up? Was it, for example, drawing and coloring, crafts, museum or gallery trips, learning handiwork from a relative, or pictures on the living room wall? Write down some notes about what you remember.
- What kind of beliefs did your family have about art?
- When you were young, did you have a favorite art or craft activity, such as coloring, painting by number, embroidering, knitting, or building things? What do you remember about it?
- Did you ever have a negative experience with art when you were a child? Were you told, for example, that you were not artistic, that your older sibling was the artist in the family, or that your art expressions were not good enough?

from fully enjoying art making in the present. When people first begin working with me in art therapy, I often ask them to complete a questionnaire that explores their personal beliefs and experiences with art. Take some time to answer the questions in the sidebar "Your Personal Art History" to clarify your own unique beliefs about art.

Becoming "Image Aware"

Identifying your image awareness is as important to discovering your beliefs about art as exploring your personal art history is. Image awareness is your awareness of the images around you—that is, what images you choose to have in your environment and how you respond to them. While art therapy emphasizes expressing images representative of the inner world of imagination and the unconscious mind, many of these are influenced by images we have around us. We all are drawn to certain colors, shapes, forms, patterns, and textures in our environment. We may consciously place them around us in decorating our home or choosing clothes to wear. We also keep in our homes or offices images and items—pictures, prints, photographs, cards, or objects—that have meaning for us, that remind us of a person, a memory, or an event, or that simply give us pleasure when we look at them.

Both your personal art history and your image awareness are reflected in your present life, particularly in your home environment. Before trying the exercises in this book, spend some time thinking about the importance of images in your life. I often ask people to tell me what images in their homes are significant to them. Do you keep photos of family and friends in your office or family room? Do you hang prints or calendars with special images on your walls? Are they pictures of nature, animals, or a certain artist's paintings that you enjoy? What objects do you like to have around you? What colors and textures do you like to have in your environment?

We all collect and place around us images that are important to us or those that have meaning or personal value. Even the colors and forms we put around us in our living areas, our workplaces, and our private spaces tell a lot about what we value. For example, in my office I keep close by a basket of hand-dyed yarns I collected in the mountains of California; pictures of family, friends, the cat, and a memorable trip to China; a large Monet print my husband purchased at a museum; a book of Georgia O'Keeffe's paintings; an assortment of plastic animals and dinosaurs that sit on the printer; a photo I took on the Atlantic coast of a large rock; a Magritte art print; and a small pile of sand dollars that I picked up on the Oregon coast. These visual images give me pleasure, help me recall gratifying and important events, and are a source of artistic inspiration. When I am going through a mental block in writing, I often use the book of O'Keeffe paintings to relax my mind. Or I enjoy the textures of the natural objects on display or rearrange (and play with) the animals and dinosaurs on my printer to escape from my projects for a few minutes.

Start by looking at what you have around you in your environment. Pick a room at home in which you keep personal images and objects. Take some time to write down a few phrases about each image or object. Try to note why you like each one. For example, perhaps you like the color or shape, or the image makes you feel happy or peaceful, or it reminds you of a particular event. In order to get the most from this experience, write down your answers, using the "Image Awareness" sidebar.

Guidelines for Drawing from Within

Before you get started on the exercises in this book, let's review some of the more important points about art therapy.

It Is Not Necessary to Be an Artist

It is not necessary to be an artist to benefit from art therapy. Don't worry about technical skills; there will be no grades and no judgments about whether your drawings or paintings are "good enough." This time you do not have to "stay within the lines."

If you think it is too late in life to get started or that you will never be creative, consider the work of Elizabeth Layton, who began to draw in her sixties without having any previous training or experience. Layton's story clearly illustrates that it is never too late to learn how to express yourself through the language of art. In working with art for self-understanding, personal growth, and health and well-being, there is no wrong way to go about it and there are no "wrong" art expressions. Layton found that taking the risk to express herself through art and trying to do the best she could were life-altering actions, ones that helped her find her way out of serious depression and profound grief.

As an art therapist and artist, I believe that all people have an innate capacity to be creative through art. In art therapy, people's worth, dignity, and self-direction are respected and supported. Part of this respect and support comes from the therapist or the environment that supports art therapy; the other part comes from the people themselves. It is important in beginning to explore yourself through art that you respect your own ability to make images and trust that you can be creative.

Trust Your Intuition

Sometimes beginning to make art is not easy because of the negative messages we have been given about art making in the past.

Image Awareness

- Pick out a part of your home or work environment where you spend most of your time. Look around at the images in that space (photos, calendars, artist prints, natural or man-made objects, cards, and so on) and make a short list of the ones that catch your eye. Notice if there are any particular colors, forms, textures, or shapes that you see within this space; list those below.
- Take some time to write down a few phrases about each image or object. Try to note why you like each one. For example, note that you like the color or shape, or the image makes you feel happy or peaceful, or it reminds you of a particular experience or event.
- What images or objects would you like to have around you that you do not see in your environment right now? Are there some that you have already but would like to have more of?
- Choose one image or object in your environment and look at it for a few minutes. Close your eyes and imagine what that image or object would look like if you could transform it into a work of art, such as a painting or sculpture. Imagine you have the capability to change its color, size, material, and texture. Note and record what that image or object would look like.

Hopefully, you have been able to identify some of these messages through the questionnaire in the earlier sidebar. To feel free to express yourself through art, you must first understand where these negative messages came from and how they inhibit you.

Art making is an intuitive process; that is, it does not depend on logic or rational thought, and it has no rules. When you use your intuition, you simply feel that you know what is right in a given situation. When engaging in any creative activity, including art making, you often use your intuition to make decisions about color, line, shape, and other qualities.

Art making involves a sense of play. Jung noted that, without play, "no creative work has ever yet come to birth." Playing generally involves feelings of pleasure, relaxation, spontaneity, exhilaration, freedom, and renewal. Play is the natural activity of children. American psychoanalyst and educator Erik Erikson, well known for his theories on human development, said that "to play it out is the most natural self-healing measure childhood affords."

Play is important to adults, too. It is behavior that enables us to feel free to explore and express without self-judgment or inhibition, to participate for the sheer joy of the experience, and to think creatively, flexibly, and innovatively. Children often expand their self-knowledge through play, using play activity to explore who they are and to understand others and their environment. For this reason, play has been called the work of children, but it is something we need throughout our lives in order to continue to learn and grow. It emphasizes the process over the result and is internally satisfying. Getting in touch with the sense of play also taps our abilities to adapt, experiment, solve problems, and change.

Being able to play means being able to communicate, to express fantasy, to overcome blocks to creativity, and to experience emotional release. To have a sense of play is extremely important to art making, especially when one is using art for therapeutic benefits.

Part of the transformative power of art is that it allows us to lose ourselves in the activity and to express previously unrealized aspects of ourselves. Trusting our intuition in making marks on paper, creating shapes in paint, or choosing colored paper for collage helps us discover new insights. Working intuitively, making art purely for the joy of creating, and making something with our own hands can also be liberating.

The Process, Not the Product, Is Important

Your immediate goal is not to produce a beautiful painting or sculpture but to express yourself, enjoy the creative process, and see what emerges. I have probably said thousands of times to art therapy clients or participants in workshops, "Don't worry if what you have created is art or not!" Let go of worries about the quality of your work and simply enjoy the process of creating.

An art experience may be therapeutic, pleasurable, or inspirational and still leave one wondering if the painting or drawing one has made is good. We all have many internal voices that form judgments about our creative work, particularly in art making, where a tangible product remains. If you find that you are repeatedly asking yourself if your work is good or correct, spend some time thinking about why you are hearing this. Write down what your inner voices say, and think about where those voices are coming from (for example, parents, partners, teachers, bosses, and so on).

There is a place for these critics, and, as an artist, I believe that there is such a thing as quality. In my own work as an artist, I know some pieces are better than others. Sometimes I find out that my husband or friends like one of my paintings that I was planning to discard. This may be a subjective feeling about quality on my part, but how you feel about your images matters in terms of self-esteem, inspiration, and motivation. In art therapy, the way an image looks is less important than the pleasure and gratification one derives from creating it—a capacity that is available to everyone in one way or another.

Do Not Analyze What You Have Created

Most of the art activities in this book ask you to be spontaneous, to put aside preconceived notions about art and art making, and to express yourself in an authentic way. Responding intuitively and with a sense of play, as described in the previous section, will help you do this. Becoming absorbed in art making is also important. In other words, try not to become distracted by what you are drawing or painting. Just allow it to take shape. Steve Nachmanovitch, author of *Free Play*, calls this disappearing. He notes that for art to appear, we often have to disappear, allowing our minds and senses to become quiet for the moment. Fully involving yourself in the activity will help you cease worrying about what your images look like and allow you to enjoy the process of creating them.

When you have finished your image, you may be tempted to try to interpret it. Part of the art therapy process involves finding personal meaning for your art expressions. Although the content of art expressions is important, the act of creating them is equally important. In getting started, try not to psychoanalyze your art for meaning and inferences. The very act of making it is a positive and transformative process. Work with the process for a while before looking at your images for meaning. Finding meaning takes time and may require the guidance of an objective observer, such as a therapist.

Writing about your work is a suggested part of each exercise in this book. Even short phrases may help you understand, over time, what your images mean to you. When you look back over both your images and your writing, patterns, connections, and new ideas will emerge. Writing about your images also serves a therapeutic purpose that is described in more detail in a later chapter.

Have an Intention

In any form of therapy, the curative process begins with the person's intention. Deciding to work on a problem is the first step toward change. A person who is working with a therapist may have already established his or her therapeutic goal. If not, the therapist may help the person develop one.

An intention is simply a plan or a purpose. In her book *Art Is a Way of Knowing*, art therapist Pat Allen notes that intention is as essential to your work as creating time and space for it. Allen says that one's intention, or goal, can be as simple as gathering the courage to experiment with materials, or it may be to deepen one's understanding of a problem one is confronting. When she begins to make art, Allen tries to formulate the clearest intention possible.

Think about what you would like to get from using art as therapy, whether you are working with the exercises in this book or with a therapist. Your intention can be as basic as exploring new experiences with drawing or painting, using art making in your life to reduce stress, or enhancing your sense of well-being through creativity. It can be to increase your understanding of how you express yourself through images or to learn more about how your feelings and life experiences are reflected in art. Your intention may change as you complete the exercises in the next couple of chapters.

Some Additional Advice About Using This Book

My overall intention for this book is to describe art therapy and how it works. Over many years of teaching the subject of art therapy to students and professionals, I have found that it is often best understood through actual experience. The art activities in the next several chapters will help the reader experience some of the ideas presented.

Although art therapy can be soothing and relaxing, art making for self-exploration can also be difficult at times. As an art therapist who uses art in my own self-exploration, personal understanding, and healing, I know that the process of art making is not always predictable. When I am in my studio painting, I am often filled with joy, but there are many other times when I am frustrated by the materials, the process, and the outcome.

If you are easily frustrated, emotionally frail, or at a point in your life where you think some psychological support would be of benefit, you may want to use the exercises in this book with your own therapist. Bring this book with you to your therapist and discuss what you would like to achieve, either by doing the exercises at home or by working on specific ones in a therapy session. Finding a professional who can work with you is a subject discussed later in this book.

While the images we create through art can be powerful and even moving, I believe that making art cannot hurt people. My two favorite T-shirts, designed by artist Fred Babb, bear the slogans "art can't hurt you" and "fear no art," underscoring art's benevolent powers. Art expression serves as a buffer between our inner and outer worlds, and images often come before we can express our thoughts and emotions in words. It is far better to get powerful images outside us in the form of art expression than to repress or contain them within. Individuals such as Elizabeth Layton and others have demonstrated that it is harmful to keep these emotions inside and that art is a healthy way to let them out.

Art making, even on one's own, has a positive effect. This effect can be enhanced by working with a professional who can help you further explore your process of art making and the content of your images. Art therapy groups and therapeutic studios are additional avenues for enhancing the depth of exploration and benefits from art making. These are also described in later chapters and in the resources section at the end of the book.

Some Limitations of Art Therapy

While doing the exercises in this book is not a substitute for working with a therapist, it will give you an idea of how art can be useful for self-exploration and personal change. Also, although art therapy is extremely versatile, it has some limitations, as does any therapeutic modality used for change.

For some people, another modality may be more enjoyable or may come more easily. Dance, music, or poetry may be more gratifying. I often ask people to use their artwork as inspiration for a poem, story, sound, or movement. Expressive therapies and creative arts therapies (music, dance, drama, writing) are not the subject of this book, but they can be more helpful than art therapy alone for some people.

While you may believe that not being naturally artistic could be a drawback, in most cases it is not. In fact, many people with formal art training who come to my practice or workshops initially have trouble being spontaneous. Artists generally have developed a style or way of working, and in art therapy they are usually asked to put that aside and make art that is not necessarily beautiful or aesthetic. Think of it this way: if you are not an artist, then you will have no preconceived notions of how your art should look.

Art therapy is not a "magic bullet." Like any process for change, it requires time, an intention to change, and active participation. While art can externalize conflicts, powerful feelings, and painful experiences, it does not automatically transform them. Modifying behavior, emotional responses, and life circumstances is often harder than transforming images in drawings and paintings.

Despite these limitations, art making can initiate a positive transformation in your life by facilitating self-exploration and self-understanding. Its power lies in the creative process, the subject of the next chapter.

4

Creativity: Drawing
on Process

*The creative process involved in the making of art is healing
and life enhancing.*

AMERICAN ART THERAPY ASSOCIATION, MISSION STATEMENT

*Everyone's creative acts, whatever they may be, make
constructive form out of the apparent formlessness of our lives.*

ROLLO MAY, *MY QUEST FOR BEAUTY*

CREATIVITY IS A means of personal growth, self-understanding,
change, and rehabilitation. Like the word *art*, creativity may bring
to mind many long-held associations. When art is mentioned, many
people think of creativity, although creative thinking is not limited
to art. Through the questionnaire in the previous chapter, you may
have identified some of your beliefs about creativity—in particular,
whether you believe yourself to be creative and how you express
yourself creatively. I believe my role as an art therapist is to help
people use art making not only for self-exploration and understanding but also for enhancing well-being.

Defining Creativity

Psychologists and scholars have had difficulty determining exactly
what creativity is and who is capable of it. They often disagree in
their definitions of creativity, some seeing it as a quality present in
all people and others believing it to be a rare gift.

Ideas about creativity, what motivates it, and who is capable of it have evolved over time. Early in the twentieth century, Freud believed that creativity originates in conflicts and that the creative process is a response to the need to solve conflicts. He considered creative works to be daydreams and fantasies in disguise—inner wishes, frustration, or discontent that is transformed into art, poetry, or music. Freud seemed to be mostly concerned with the motivation for creativity and less with the essence of the creative process itself.

Jung, on the other hand, believed that the creative process occurs in two modes: psychological and visionary. In the psychological mode, the content of art, poetry, or music comes from the realm of human consciousness—what we see around us in reality. The visionary mode of creativity concerned Jung more deeply. He believed that this mode of creativity comes from our depths, what Jung called the collective unconscious, or the place where archetypes reside. Jung believed the greatness of a creative work resulted from the reactivation of an archetype through an art form such as painting, literature, or music. A truly remarkable creative work transcends life experiences and often has universal meaning. In Jung's view, creativity is seen as a great gift held by geniuses, those capable of the visionary mode of expression. By this definition, artists such as Leonardo da Vinci, Michelangelo, and Pablo Picasso had the qualities necessary for creative work. They produced art that transcended life and generated universal responses from its viewers.

Since the time of Freud and Jung, we have come to believe that creativity is available to everyone. It is a quality shared by all of us, to a greater or lesser extent. Howard Gardner, a developmental psychologist, makes a distinction between creativity with a big *C* and creativity with a little *c*. Big C creativity is responsible for accomplishments such as social progress, the development of civilization, or the creation of an artistic masterpiece. But we all regularly use creative skills to modify thinking, to solve problems, to create beauty or aesthetic appeal, and to make everyday life special. This is *little c creativity*, our personal creativity that is used to enhance life and provide satisfaction. Many aspects of daily life involve some form of this type of creativity: arranging flowers in a vase, setting a colorful table, or designing a plan for a vegetable garden. I often ask people about the creative acts in their daily lives, helping them see that they are already using imagination and creativity to enhance their surroundings and create pleasure through images in their environment for themselves and others. In this broader sense, we are all creative.

Creativity is often defined as the ability to bring something new and unique into existence; as a union of opposites, impressions, ideas, and concepts that initially seem unrelated; or as giving birth to a new idea. Although these definitions explain the creative process, it is more easily understood when you think about its qualities and characteristics, rather than an overarching definition. Creativity is thought to include many or all of the following qualities: spontaneity, playfulness, imagination, motivation, originality, self-expression, inventiveness, divergent thinking, and intuition. Creative people are known to be more independent, autonomous, self-sufficient, emotionally sensitive, assertive, self-accepting (particularly of the irrational parts of themselves), resourceful, adventurous, and risk taking.

Creativity is a form of pushing limits, inventing, breaking down boundaries, and rejecting accepted assumptions. During a creative moment you begin to recognize the limitations of your present way of thinking or ways of looking at the world. You let go of old beliefs and perceptions. In this sense, creativity, as Rollo May pointed out, takes a great deal of courage. In art making or any activity other than an imitative one, the courage to create something new and unique can provide a sense of satisfaction and personal involvement that makes it meaningful and worthwhile.

Over the past several decades, creativity has come to be defined as a human potential, a capacity we can develop in ourselves if we want to. In his book *On Becoming a Person*, psychologist Carl Rogers observed that "the mainspring of creativity appears to be the same tendency which we discover so deeply as the curative force in psychotherapy—man's tendency to actualize himself, to become his potentialities." Humanistic psychologists such as Rogers emphasize the importance of creativity, play, and spontaneity in human potential. They consider the creative process to be part of our ability to self-actualize. Self-actualization enables us to make life more meaningful, to enhance our abilities, to know ourselves, and to reach our full potential.

Understanding the Creative Process

Despite years of research on creativity and the creative process, we still do not know exactly how creative breakthroughs result. While there are many theories about the creative process, most generally include the following stages:

1. Preparation (gathering materials and ideas)
2. Incubation (becoming absorbed in the process)
3. Illumination (experiencing a breakthrough and achievement)
4. Verification (adding final touches or making changes)

These stages commonly describe the creative process used in a variety of endeavors, from simple problem solving to more lofty activities such as making a scientific discovery or completing a painting, musical piece, or poem.

Because the creative process involved in visual art is a hands-on experience that involves both the mind and the senses, it is also thought to involve other unique aspects. Art therapist Vija Lusebrink observes that artistic creativity includes a number of experiences, including kinesthetic/sensory (action), perceptual/affective (form), and cognitive/symbolic (image).

On a *kinesthetic/sensory level*, an individual has to interact with art materials in an exploratory way that is characterized by movement; motor activity; and tactile, visual, and other senses. At this level, the actual details of what is created are not important; what's important is the body's experience of sensory expression through art materials. On the *perceptual/affective level*, an individual engages with art materials to communicate ideas and emotions. At this level, one is able to convey feeling or perception through art expression. On the *cognitive/symbolic level*, a person uses art materials to convey personal meaning through structure, elaboration, and modification of form and image. In other words, the art maker uses materials to create a personal symbol to communicate feelings, thoughts, or events.

According to Lusebrink, the fourth level—the creative level—is an integration of all other levels within an art form. Not all individuals reach this level, but a form of creativity can be encountered at each of the three other levels. For example, an individual can experience creativity through using colors and lines to express an emotion in paint (perceptual/affective), through simply moving a pencil across the paper (kinesthetic/sensory), or through developing an image that symbolizes a concept or an idea (cognitive/symbolic). When all of these levels come together in a drawing, painting, or sculpture, the product becomes truly creative, unique, and evocative to viewers.

Most importantly personal variations exist in how the creative process of art making is experienced by each individual. These variations are important to the process of art therapy. Personal creativity depends a great deal on your interest level in the activity in which you are engaged and whether that activity is meaningful to you and personally motivating. When trying the activities in this book, you will find some more inspiring and gratifying than others and may feel more comfortable with certain media. Discovering your preferences for materials and activities will ultimately help you to find and nurture your creative potential and stimulate your creative juices.

Art Therapy and the Creative Process

The guiding principle behind art therapy is stated in the beginning of this chapter: "the creative process involved in the making of art is healing and life enhancing." The fact that this idea is integral to art therapy is not surprising because there are many similarities between the creative process and the process of therapy. Both creativity and art therapy are about solving problems—finding new solutions to old ways of being, thinking, feeling, and interacting. The creative process, like the therapeutic process, also provides an opportunity to explore and experiment with new ideas and ways of being. Both processes are acts of modification, alteration, improvisation, and transformation. In therapy, these characteristics are essential to creating new understanding, insight, and awareness—preludes to making changes in oneself, one's perceptions, and one's life. Both involve an encounter with self; in art therapy, this encounter is through art materials and the art-making experience.

Art therapist and colleague Lori Vance's work embodies the characteristics in her creative process with mixed media. She rearranges and alters collage elements, combining them with paint or drawing and natural objects. A fragment of a photo image of a flower is transformed into a heart; and a bar code, a postage stamp, or feathers become inventive parts of the composition (Figures 4.1, 4.2, and 4.3).

Lori pushes limits in how she uses materials in her artworks and demonstrates that the creative process of art making offers the unique opportunity to take what is familiar and even ordinary, explore new ways of working with images, engage one's sense of play, and encounter oneself in the process. Taking what she learns from her own artistic creativity into her work as an art therapist, Lori helps adolescents and adults explore themselves, take risks through new behaviors, and encounter themselves through visual arts, drumming, and creative movement. In my mind, she embodies the potential of the creative process to transform oneself and to encourage personal transformation in others.

In art therapy, you are asked to use your creativity to make original and imaginative artwork. It is not an imitative experience in

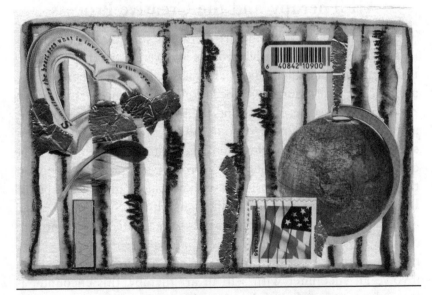

Figure 4.1 *Attending to the Pain*, a mixed-media collage by Lori Vance
(Reprinted with permission of the artist)

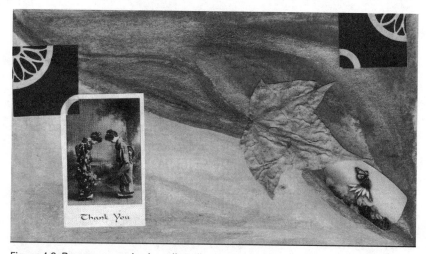

Figure 4.2 *Reverence*, a mixed-media collage by Lori Vance
(Reprinted with permission of the artist)

which you are asked to follow a series of directions, copy an image, or learn how to be technically proficient. Successfully replicating a craft project or duplicating a drawing or sculpture may provide you with a sense of satisfaction, but it does not take you through a creative process in which you discover and develop your own personal

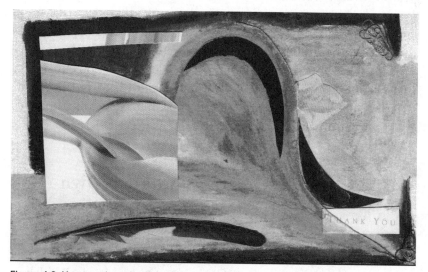

Figure 4.3 *Heartseed*, a mixed-media collage by Lori Vance
(Reprinted with permission of the artist)

and authentic imagery. Working with your own image-making process and taking the risk of expressing yourself without judgment connects you to your creative potential.

Ultimately, art therapy is a process that involves exploring, modifying, and creating images, working from your own imagination, and often going into the unknown. This can be unnerving at times, especially when you are just beginning. In tapping your creative source, there are no models to follow and no examples to copy or reproduce. Creativity inevitably involves taking risks, breaking boundaries, pushing limits, and inventing new ideas. If you feel secure with rules and with getting the right answer, this experience will probably initially feel frustrating, contradictory, and perhaps exasperating. While it is not always an easy experience, art therapy is worth pursuing because it can be the beginning of personal change, growth, and integration. It can lead to insight, self-awareness, and transformation—common goals in most forms of therapy and healing.

Lori Vance's work also demonstrates that true creativity is playful, spontaneous, and imaginative. It frees you to make your own rules and, in the process of doing so, often breaks down previously held assumptions. Her mixed-media pieces exemplify a key characteristic of the creative process that is strongly connected to emotional health: divergent thinking. Divergent thinking is an experience of moving beyond perceived limits; synthesizing and integrating unrelated elements; and reorganizing or altering previously accepted thoughts, ideas, and perceptions. Immersing yourself in the creative process of art therapy is, in its simplest sense, a hands-on experience that encourages you to think divergently and to try out new perspectives and ways of thinking in order to enhance and nurture your emotional health.

Promoting Creativity in Your Own Art Making

Before you try the art therapy exercises described later in this book, it is helpful to explore your personal definition of creativity. As you answer the questions in the "Creativity Questionnaire" sidebar,

Creativity Questionnaire

1. How do you define creativity?
2. Do you consider yourself a creative person? If you do, what characteristics make you creative? If you do not, why not? Who in your life do you consider creative? What characteristics make this person creative?
3. Can you recall an instance in which you were particularly creative? Describe that instance.
4. Are there cycles to your creativity? Are there times when you are more creative than others?
5. Is there something in particular that inspires your creativity? Are you more creative when you are happy, or does some other emotion drive your creativity? Do you feel more creative working alone or in a group?
6. How do you feel when you are not creative?
7. Is there a creative activity you want to pursue but have been postponing? What is it? What is stopping you from doing it? Is there a creative project that you started but never finished?

think about what circumstances help you feel creative, what distracts you from creative pursuits, and what you would like to create, particularly if it's something you've been putting off.

For all the definitions of creativity, there are just as many theories about how to promote it. While creativity is not something that can be taught, there are conditions that can support it. Following are some of the more common ones.

A "Permissive" Attitude

Creativity flourishes where there are no judgments, preconceptions, or biases. To express yourself creatively, you must feel free to try new experiences, break rules and assumptions, and play freely with ideas. It is OK to tear the paper, to destroy and rearrange your images, and to create your own unique way of working with materials. You do not have to follow whatever rules you may have been taught or imitate the way others draw or paint.

Humanistic psychologist Carl Rogers observed that creativity is closely associated with one's openness to experiences. To be creative, we must put aside preconceived notions and take in new information and situations. In other words, the ability to tolerate ambiguity and contradictory information is key to the creative process.

Lack of Fear or Concern About What Others Might Think

As noted in Chapter 3, it is important to simply trust the process and follow your instincts and intuition. Creativity flourishes when we have an inner sense of knowing what is right for ourselves, not when we rely on the praise or judgments of others. Ask yourself these questions: Is the process satisfying for me? Do my images express my feelings and thoughts? When you are creating for yourself and without concern for what others may think, these questions are the ones that really matter. It may also be time to let go of some of the negative beliefs that you discovered through the questions in the "Creativity Questionnaire" sidebar.

Letting Go of Self-Criticism

In order to feel free to experiment and explore, you must let go of inner voices that say things like "Be careful," "Don't waste paint," or "You should be doing something else" (for example, the laundry, sorting the papers on your desk, or changing the oil in the car). An important gift to yourself in art making is to allow yourself the freedom to explore and experiment without worrying about how or how many materials you use or how much time you spend in the process.

In addition, in using your creative resources for self-exploration and self-expression, don't worry about whether you are making something "useful." Your purpose is simply to create and enjoy the activity.

Acceptance That There Is No Right or Wrong Answer

This requires setting aside rules about right and wrong and treating one's perceived errors with respect, because out of these often come new insights. Making an accidental line in a drawing or spilling the paint across the paper can lead to new discoveries and unexpected results.

Developing an Intention and a Passion

Developing your creativity through art making does take commitment. The saying "Creativity is 5 percent inspiration and 95 percent perspiration" is true. Working at something intentionally and with passion unlocks the creative process. You have to be willing to commit to the process, to stay with it, and to trust that it will unfold exactly as it should.

Relaxation and Creativity

Creativity comes from many sources within and is encouraged by many factors in our surroundings. Outwardly, we may need an environment for art making, materials, a sense of safety, and a climate of acceptance. Inwardly, creativity may come from excitement, exhilaration, and inspiration and, at other times, from more peaceful and deeper places within ourselves. Solitude, inactivity, and daydreaming are all states of being that encourage creativity. These are all times when we are in a relaxed state of consciousness, times when creativity can flow naturally, and when our minds are most receptive to images.

Shaun McNiff, in his book *Trust the Process*, observes that artists are able to step aside from their work and relax in order to make new discoveries. They work with the creative process, encouraging it either forcefully or subtly, but are always respectful of what takes shape outside the sphere of their control. They are willing to let go, relax, and trust that something will emerge.

As I mentioned earlier, "letting go" is often necessary in the process of art therapy, and many people find it helpful to completely relax before they begin art making. This is a matter of personal preference and is not essential to do before beginning the exercises in this book. However, relaxation can help you become more focused and release some of the tension, assumptions, or preconceptions that you have. I often start work sessions with a short relaxation exercise. Many people find it helpful to relax before art making in order to establish a transition between the events of the day and time for personal creativity.

The following exercise is commonly used in stress reduction and relaxation. You may want to tape-record it so that you can listen to it rather than having to memorize it. Before beginning, sit in a comfortable chair, with your legs uncrossed. If you are sitting at a table, you may rest your arms on the tabletop or let them drop to your lap.

1. Close your eyes and focus on your breath, slowly inhaling and exhaling three times.
2. Continue to inhale and exhale slowly and relax the muscles in your face, especially the area around your jaw. Let your jaw open slightly, so that any tension there can flow away from your face.
3. Relax the muscles in your scalp and neck, letting your head move forward slightly.
4. Relax the muscles in your shoulders and, from there, let the relaxation move down into the muscles of your arms and hands. Continue to feel the tension slip away from your back, over your chest, down to your stomach, and all the way down to the base of your spine.
5. Let the feeling of relaxation spread to your thighs, knees, and lower legs, down to your ankles and feet until it reaches the tips of your toes.
6. Start from the top of your head and work down. Take a few moments now to scan your body for any part that is not fully relaxed. If you feel any part of your body that is

not fully relaxed, take a deep breath and send the breath into that area, imagining warmth and relaxation reaching it. When you exhale, imagine the tension leaving your body with the breath.

A variation that I find relaxing is to imagine inhaling a colored mist or light. You can choose any color that feels comfortable or relaxing to you. That color can also become an inspiration for the art that you make after you complete the relaxation exercise.

An alternative to a relaxation exercise may be simply to play some calming music. The type of music you play is again a personal preference. Meditation often employs classical, instrumental, or percussion pieces, and you may find these calming. You may want to try a relaxation exercise in conjunction with the exercises in the next chapter on spontaneous imagery.

Getting into the Flow

The creative process can be a particularly fulfilling experience when you are able to become so engrossed in an activity that you actually lose track of time. Mihaly Csikszentmihalyi describes this experience as flow, a unique state of concentration when you feel positive and energized, focused, and totally absorbed in the present moment. In sports, this is what is often referred to as reaching the zone, a physical and mental state of transcendence. Everything around you except the task at hand is forgotten while awareness and action become one.

Daniel Goleman, an expert on behavioral and brain sciences, observes that flow is emotional intelligence at its best. Emotional intelligence includes self-awareness of one's feelings, self-motivation, and empathy for the emotional experience of others. Goleman believes that emotional intelligence is essential for creativity and is an ability one can cultivate through being in flow. During the flow state, people are more productive because they are focused, calm, and self-satisfied. Like the experience of meditation, brain waves are actually in a state of relaxed alertness that facilitates inspiration and confidence. If you are painting, drawing, or constructing while in a flow state, you may feel like you are part of or one with your creation.

While you may already have experienced flow in your own life, the following suggestions can help you experience it through art making to enhance your creative potential.

- **Challenge yourself.** The flow state occurs when you engage in an activity that stretches your abilities but is not so difficult that you become discouraged or bored. In other words, choose a creative activity and then engage in it at a level slightly above your ability.
- **Maintain your focus.** Stay in the present moment and do not judge how you are performing or what you are creating. As discussed in Chapter 3, just allow whatever you are working on to take shape and let yourself disappear. Anxiety prevents flow, so try a relaxation exercise like the one in the previous section, or play baroque music in the background—the tempo of 60 to 70 beats per minute naturally induces a state of relaxed alertness.
- **Give yourself time.** An important ingredient of creativity is time. If you have to work creative expression into your schedule, try to give yourself enough time so that you are not torn away from the experience of deep concentration. Repeatedly stopping in the middle of what you love to do and from the experience of flow more than anything will stifle creativity.
- **Allow yourself to become hooked.** Once you find flow through a creative activity, return to it whenever you can. The more you experience this blissful state, the more you will want to return to it. And the more you return to it, the easier you will "go with the flow" and find deeper satisfaction in the creative process.

Before moving on, it is important to understand that becoming more creative is not a panacea for emotional difficulties, personal conflicts, family problems, or lack of life satisfaction. However, creativity does have a powerful influence on personality, providing an opportunity for experimentation, exploration, and discovery, moving beyond limits, finding inner resources, and realizing your own potential for change and growth. The creative process of art making can create a sense of self-esteem and self-assurance, increase sensitivity and understanding of yourself, and enhance your overall quality of life.

5

Setting Up: Drawing on Environment and Materials

Dealing with the inherent beauty of materials and their
unfailing reliability can involve us in a deeply healing process.

JOAN M. ERIKSON,
WISDOM AND THE SENSES: THE WAY OF CREATIVITY

ART THERAPY INVOLVES more than learning to trust the creative process and drawing from within. It also requires knowing how to create an appropriate environment and understanding how art materials promote a wide range of expression. When you're working with a therapist, the environment and materials are usually provided. Many therapists encourage people to use simple materials in order to stimulate spontaneous expression. The emphasis is on using materials to quickly create an image that can be used to initiate a verbal exchange between the person and the therapist.

In my own practice as an art therapist, I am interested in helping people learn more about the materials with which they will work. I believe that knowing what art materials can do helps people develop their visual language and deepens their experience of art therapy. I usually ask people to continue their art making at home, so I consider it important to advise people on how to choose art materials and how to set up a space at home in which to work. I like to introduce people to more complex materials, especially if they want to expand beyond simple drawing and painting activities. If you are trying some of the art therapy exercises described in this book, it is also important that you know more about materials and how to create a workable space in which to make art.

Creating a Space

An environment conducive to creativity is an important part of art therapy. When you are working with a therapist, you may find yourself in an office or a studio, depending on the therapist. Some therapists' offices have a table or an easel for art making or expressive work, while others have studio space similar to what an artist might have. Art therapists who work in hospitals or clinics may have elaborate art rooms in which to work with people either individually or in groups. If they work with people who are disabled or confined by illness to beds or rooms, they may have to adapt the space for art activities.

It is nice to have a room that is completely devoted to creative activities, but often this is not possible. However, even the smallest and simplest of spaces can be transformed into an art area. When I work with children in shelters, often I have to adapt a kitchen table (and sometimes a Ping-Pong table) or part of the TV room into an art-making area. People in hospitals or nursing homes must often work at their bedside or on their tray tables. As limited as these small environments seem, it is always possible to create an area suitable for art making.

Most of the exercises in this book do not require a great deal of space, and some are even portable (visual journals, for example). However, it is essential to have some space at home where you can set out your materials, work comfortably, and leave art in progress. Working on your own may take some thought about where to make art and how you can fit it into your circumstances and lifestyle. If you will be working on the art experientials in this book at home, you will need to identify a space where you can actually make art. The following factors are important to consider when selecting and setting up a space for your art making.

Environment

Having a special room for art making is optimal but not always necessary, especially when you are just beginning. There is probably a place in your home where you can work—perhaps a corner of a room, a basement, or an all-purpose room. You may have to rearrange some furniture or set up a folding screen to partition off a space.

It is ideal to have a space in which you can leave materials set up for use, as well as works in progress, such as wet paintings or unfinished collages. If it isn't possible to have such a place in your home, it is important that you keep materials in one place and ready to use. It is also crucial to have a place where you can feel at ease making a mess. Try to choose a place where you can leave works in progress instead of having to dismantle and put away your work each time.

Surface

You may feel comfortable working on the floor, but most people need a tabletop to work on. If this is not possible, you may want to purchase a drawing board or a smooth piece of plywood that you can balance on your lap or lay across another surface. Some people use their kitchen tables for art making, but be sure that your surface isn't cluttered with the toaster, condiments, or other items that can distract you or get in the way. When choosing a surface to work at, you will want to pick one that will be just for art making, if possible.

An easel is another alternative. There are simple, inexpensive table easels that can hold a board so that you can work on an upright surface. Some people prefer to work on a wall, tacking or fastening their paper to the wall. In my own studio, I have an old smooth-surfaced door that I can lean against the wall and slide behind furniture when not in use. If you have a wall on which you would like to work, you might try attaching a drywall board to the wall. You can paint it white (or a color to match your wall) and tack paper or other materials to it. This type of work area can also serve as a place in which to hang completed works or works in progress.

You may want to protect your work surface with a piece of heavy paper or cardboard if you are concerned about damage.

Storage

If the area you are working in serves more than one purpose (for example, the kitchen table or a portion of your family room), it is helpful to have some storage containers to hold your supplies. Cardboard boxes or tin candy containers can hold drawing and painting supplies, and simple plastic crates are good for paper, sketchbooks, and larger items.

A basket with compartments to hold a sketchbook and drawing materials, scissors, glue, and a few other simple supplies can be helpful if you want to work away from home. Although I have a studio space in which I can paint and create, I keep a picnic basket filled with paper, drawing tools, and other supplies so that I can carry it into other rooms or spaces. Your art basket can go with you to parks, waiting rooms, your car, or other people's homes.

Light

Natural light is best but not always available. Simple desk lamps are a good alternative; they can be adjusted in various directions, are inexpensive, and can be found at most department stores. Many desk lamps attach to a table with a screw-on device. Avoid fluorescent light, which is hard on your eyes.

Exhibition

A place to hang up your work where you can see it is important and can be as simple as a wall or bulletin board. The drywall boards mentioned in the previous section are also good for display. Seeing your images can help motivate you and lead you to think of new ideas and directions.

Safety

It is also important to have a sense of trust and safety within the space you choose to make art. This may mean a space that affords privacy and where your work is safe from damage.

In my work with children who have been abused or exposed to domestic violence, I try to create an atmosphere where all art expression is unconditionally acceptable. A nonjudgmental stance is essential if these traumatized children are to feel free to express themselves.

When working with adults who come to art therapy because of issues of trauma and loss, emotional difficulties, or family problems, I am also cognizant of their feelings of trust and safety. Like many of you reading this book, they may have initial doubts or anxieties about art making, fearing failure or embarrassment or simply not knowing where to begin. As an art therapist, I try to convey the ideas previously mentioned: it is not necessary that they be trained artists; the process is what is important; they should trust their own intuition and way of working; and they should not worry about what they have created.

If you are trying the exercises in this book on your own, you won't necessarily have the benefit of a reflective and supportive person to guide and encourage you. In this case, it is important to consider how you can make the space in which you are working feel safe and conducive to your own creative process. For some people, privacy is crucial during art making; for others, respect for their art expressions, materials, and working space is necessary.

Personal Preferences

Depending on your preferences, windows, fresh air, or aesthetic objects such as plants or furnishings may be necessary to stimulate your creativity. Sometimes music is helpful to set the mood or to help you relax and focus on what you are doing. The type of music is a matter of personal preference. Many people enjoy working to classical or instrumental music; you might want to experiment with different types of music to see what stimulates your creativity.

Time

Be sure that your workplace can be used without distraction for extended periods of time. You also need to make a personal commitment to allow yourself enough time to make art; this is part of having a personal intention, an element discussed in Chapters 3 and 4. You have to be willing to set aside enough uninterrupted time to completely immerse yourself in the creative process.

General Advice on Gathering Art Materials and Supplies

If you see a professional art therapist, art materials will usually be supplied, and your therapist will show you how they work. I believe that people must become familiar with such materials in order to have the best possible art therapy experience. Knowing materials helps you to understand what different materials can do and provides a foundation for exploration through art.

If you have not used art materials before, you may be surprised that each has its own "personality." A pencil, a piece of chalk, a crayon, and a felt marker can all be used in drawing, but each has very different characteristics. Paper also can have many different qualities, from very smooth to porous to rough.

Art therapists sometimes design art-making activities for their clients based on the characteristics of certain materials. For instance, some media are more fluid (for example, watercolors, tempera or acrylic paints, or chalk pastels). These materials are easier to manipulate but harder to control because they are watery (such as paints) or powdery (such as chalk pastels). Some media, in contrast, are considered to be more resistive (for example, pencils, felt-tip markers, and cut-paper collage). These materials permit you to be more precise and detailed, and they are easier to control.

In my work with children who have emotional difficulties or have experienced trauma, I often consider how materials affect them. For example, with children who are very emotional or hyperactive, I may guide them toward materials that are less fluid and more controlled, such as collage, or toward drawing with felt-tip markers. In choosing more resistive materials, I am trying to provide them with a more structured experience and reduce their anxiety or energy level to a calmer state. On other occasions, I might guide them toward more fluid materials, such as paint or soft clay. For example, I have worked with many children who have been traumatized by abuse or neglect and who have lost their ability to be playful or are timid or restrained in expressing themselves. In this situation, I might choose to give them materials such as paint in order to help them loosen up, play, and freely express themselves. These are two rather simple examples that describe how an art therapist might think about materials. When you are working with materials specified for the activities in this book, be aware that they do indeed have various qualities that are important in terms of art making and will have an impact on the art you make.

It also may be helpful to think of the qualities of art materials as part of a continuum. Art therapist Helen Landgarten developed a way of classifying materials from more controlled to least controlled. For example, lead and colored pencils are on the most controlled end of the continuum, because they are more resistive and you can control detail and precision. Wet materials such as wet clay and watercolors—media that are less easy to contain and control—are on the other end of the chart.

As you start to work with art materials through the exercises in this book, you may find that you have a preference for one material over another. You may like the fluidity of paint over the more resistive qualities of colored pencils, or you may prefer the tactile qualities of collage or clay. Size is also a factor. Some days you may like to work on large white paper, while other days a two-inch square will seem right. You may also find over time that you change your preferences for media or that a new material helps you feel more creative and personally satisfied than another. There is no right or wrong answer about which materials are best to use; just keep experimenting with them, and you will discover what works for you.

In addition, art materials are available in a fairly wide range of prices, and your first trip to an art supply store may be a little overwhelming for that reason. Take your time, stop to touch and feel materials, and ask questions when you are confused. If you are intimidated with the thought of going to an art store, there are alternatives that are less threatening and often less expensive. Many discount department stores have a small arts-and-crafts section stocked with economical sketchbooks, drawing materials, and paints. Office supply warehouses also may have materials at a reasonable price. Another alternative is an art supply catalog. (There are several mail-order companies listed in the resources section that have the materials you will need to complete the exercises in this book.)

You can also collect or salvage free materials. Start to save colorful magazines, catalogs, cards, and other paper that you would normally throw away. You may also want to save interesting shopping bags, boxes, lids, and containers; these items will be useful in your collage box (discussed later in this chapter), both as art materials and as sources of inspiration.

Examining Specific Types of Drawing Surfaces and Materials

Before you get started with the exercises in this book, gather the materials you will need. The following section lists basic materials and outlines their qualities. I often give people who come to art therapy a similar list to help them become acquainted with art supplies for use at home and as a resource to take with them to the art store.

By *drawing surface*, I mean anything on which you can draw. Paper (discussed in the next section) is the most familiar drawing surface, but there are others. You actually can draw on or with just about anything, because drawing is not just limited to pencil and paper. You may remember as a child drawing with a stick in the sand or mud or looking up at the sky and tracing clouds with your fingers. While you were not using pencils and paper, these are still experiences of drawing and of making lines, patterns, shapes, and designs.

Paper

It is important to have good quality paper on which to draw or paint. The most economical paper you can buy is newsprint. Newsprint is lightweight and very inexpensive and comes in a variety of sizes. It comes either in pads or rolls, the latter of which you can sometimes get from newspaper companies for free or at minimal cost. It may have either a smooth or a rough texture and is generally used for sketching with pencils or charcoal. It does not stand up to sharp pencils, which may cut through it, and will not take paint because water weakens it very easily. However, a 14 × 17 inch pad is good to have on hand for experimenting with materials such as pencils, crayons, markers, or pastels.

Buy a sketchbook or drawing pad with eighty-pound white paper for multipurpose drawing and collage work. These come in a variety of sizes and have different types of bindings. In the beginning, you may prefer a spiral-bound sketchbook because it lies flat and is the easiest to work with. You can also have a local photocopy store make a very economical spiral-bound sketchbook for you out of 8½ × 11 inch paper. Standard photocopy paper is fine for the drawing exercises in this book and some of the collage exercises, too, but it will not stand up to paint and other materials.

Artist Journals

In addition to sketchbooks and drawing pads, a variety of artist journals, nicely bound books with white drawing paper inside, can be found at both variety stores and art stores. They come in many different sizes, from small enough to keep in a pocket or handbag to very large. It is good to have a couple of sizes on hand; like paper, you may prefer one over another because of size.

Most journals and sketch pads are rectangular in shape, but some are square; you may want to purchase one of the latter to do some of the exercises in this book, particularly for the mandala drawing journal, which will be described in Chapter 6. You can also take papers that you like (white or colored) and have them cut to the size you prefer and bound at most photocopy stores.

Butcher Paper and Kraft Paper

Butcher paper is white and comes in rolls of various widths, anywhere from 24 to 54 inches. You can buy it by the foot for very little money at office supply and art stores. While you may want to use it for individual projects, it is often used in art therapy for group work where a large format is needed.

Kraft paper is similar to butcher paper, but it is generally sturdier and comes in many colors. You might want to try a few large pieces of brown kraft paper for collage work or if you want to work in a format larger than a sketchbook.

Other Drawing Surfaces

When I was a starving artist in art school, I could not always afford the best drawing paper and was forced to find many materials other than standard drawing pads or papers on which to make drawings. Paper grocery bags were one of my favorite materials to scavenge from friends and trash barrels; I especially liked the ones that were wrinkled and worn. Now that I can afford most types of paper, there are still many days when I prefer to draw on old paper bags, the backs of business cards, a pad of adhesive notes, a manila folder, or the inside of an old envelope. Both size and texture are important qualities, and sometimes I like to draw with a ballpoint pen on a small square notepad, while other times I am attracted to the surface and size of a large brown paper grocery bag. All of these are possibilities for creative work; keep a large folder or box handy to save papers, bags, folders, and cards that could be possible drawing surfaces in the future.

Oil Pastels

Oil pastels (for example, Cray-Pas) are soft, greasy drawing sticks that come in a variety of colors and are a very easy material with which to work. You can buy inexpensive sets of oil pastels at an art store; large department stores often carry them, too. They are good to use in most drawings where you want to blend or mix colors.

Chalk Pastels

Chalk pastels come in sticks and are powdery, like blackboard chalk. They are similar to oil pastels in that you can blend them and create soft edges and lines. They can be a bit messy because of the dust, so be careful to use them in a place where you don't have to worry about the colored chalk dust getting on furniture. You should also use a fixative after completing a drawing to prevent it from smudging. You can use hairspray or an artist's spray fixative. The latter can be very toxic and should only be used outdoors or in a room with adequate ventilation.

Chalk pastels come in sets. A set of twelve or twenty-four colors is a good assortment to start with.

Artists' Pencils

It is important to have a couple of good artists' pencils on hand for general sketching or making drawings. A regular number 2 pencil will do for the activities in this book, but I usually encourage people to get a couple of drawing pencils from an art store, too. The pencils you buy there come in degrees of hardness and softness. For example, a number 1 is much harder and makes lighter lines than a number 6, which is very soft and makes very dark lines. Number 2, 4, and 6 pencils are a good selection; if you like to make very dark lines, also buy an ebony pencil. In addition, be sure to pick up a couple of good erasers. (Don't rely on the one on the end of your yellow office pencil.)

Felt-Tip Markers

Felt-tip markers are readily available and easy to work with. Their only real drawback is permanence; that is, you cannot erase what you have drawn. The positive side is that they come in a wide range of brilliant colors and can be particularly stimulating and fun to work with.

Markers can have either fine or broad tips. If you like to draw with markers, be sure to get some of both types. Fine tips are good for drawing details, while broad ones are useful for coloring in large areas. You will find both types sold in boxed sets and individually. When buying markers, you should at least have one of each of the colors in the spectrum (red, orange, yellow, green, blue, purple), plus black and brown. Felt-tip markers are one material where price makes a substantial difference in quality. The cheaper ones have a limited color range, they dry out rapidly, and their tips wear quickly and break easily. A good compromise is to buy some of the less expensive ones and supplement them with a few more expensive markers in your favorite colors.

Paint

All the paints suggested for use in this book are water soluble. In other words, you can clean your hands and painting instruments in water and mild soap, such as dishwashing liquid. When you're starting to use paint and set up a painting space, it is easier to use water-soluble paints than oils, which require additional paint thinners and cleaning supplies. Water-soluble paints do not give off strong odors like oil paints do; this is important if ventilation is a problem or if you are sensitive to chemical smells.

Watercolor paints, which are easy to find at department and art stores, come in tubes and trays. You may be familiar with the eight-color watercolor sets that children use in school. A simple set of tray watercolors will do quite a bit, especially if you use watercolor paper and a good brush. Tube colors come in sets, or you can buy single tubes at some stores, and they are available in a wide range of colors. Watercolors are suited to spontaneous images because they are less easily controlled and can be blended easily with water.

Tempera paints come in a variety of colors and are very fluid and easy to use. You can purchase very small jars in sets at large department stores and larger bottles at school supply stores. You may remember using powdered tempera paints as a child. Buying powdered tempera is a less expensive option, but expect a lot of dust when you are mixing the powder with water. It is better to buy tempera in jars to save yourself breathing in the dust and the mess of mixing them.

Acrylic paints are fast drying, generally opaque, and very easy to use. They come in tubes or jars, and most are nontoxic, although it is important to check the label when in doubt. They were developed as an alternative to oil paints, which take a long time to dry and have an odor that may be a problem in a small space. You can find acrylic paints in beginner's paint sets at art stores in a standard selection of colors, which can be mixed with each other to create additional colors.

All paints require brushes. Buy relatively good brushes if you can, because they will last a long time and you will be happier with them. Finding that the bristles or hairs of cheap brushes keep falling out and sticking to your painting is a frustrating experience. Try to buy one or two good watercolor brushes and a couple of synthetic flat and round brushes for acrylic paints and tempera. Also, buy several foam brushes. They are very durable, come in various sizes, and can be used with acrylics and tempera paints. Foam brushes come in handy when you want to cover a large area with paint, and they are easy to clean. You can purchase these at any department or hardware store.

Gesso

Gesso is a white creamy painting medium used to prime surfaces such as canvas for painting. It is suggested for some of the experientials in this book when painting is required. It is good to have at least a quart of it on hand. You can use gesso on a variety of materials to create surfaces for painting, including cardboard, wood, metal, or plastic. For example, gesso can be useful if you want to paint a plastic box; a thin layer of gesso will prepare the surface for painting or collage.

A simple and inexpensive surface on which to paint can be easily made with gesso and cardboard. Save some corrugated cardboard boxes, cut them into flat sections, and cover the surfaces with gesso. I also use gesso on lightweight shirt cardboard and inexpensive watercolor paper (see next section) as substitutes for more expensive canvases. If you do several at one time, you will have a variety of sizes of surfaces on which to work when you are ready to paint.

Watercolor Paper

Although the exercises in this book do not require watercolor paper, you may want to try some for painting. Regular sketchbook paper can be used for watercolor, but it often is too flimsy for paint and cannot withstand brushwork and water.

Watercolor paper is thicker than regular paper and has a porous quality that accepts paint readily. There are various kinds of watercolor paper, defined by their surfaces: cold press (slightly textured), hot press (smooth), and rough (heavily textured). Watercolor paper generally comes in a block of ten or fifteen sheets; you remove each sheet after you have finished a painting. You can also buy watercolor paper by the sheet.

You might want to try an inexpensive watercolor block or purchase several sheets of student-grade watercolor paper. As mentioned in the preceding section, you can coat student-grade watercolor paper with gesso and use it for acrylic or tempera painting.

Collage

Collage involves adhering papers, found objects, or other materials onto a flat surface, such as heavy paper, cardboard, or wood. Common materials for collage include newspapers, magazine pictures, tissue paper, fabric, and string, as well as found materials, such as grasses, tree bark, shells, twigs, and other natural objects.

Collage is a popular modality for art therapy because it appeals to people who are intimidated by drawing or painting. For a simple paper collage, all you need is a variety of textural papers and a sturdy surface to which you can attach them. Paper is also one of the easiest materials with which to work and requires very simple tools and supplies—a good pair of scissors, white glue or rubber cement, and a variety of papers and found objects. You can cut or tear papers to use in a collage and include anything else that will adhere to the surface.

Use a small cardboard packing box to collect pictures from magazines and catalogs, junk mail, stamps, grocery wrappers, wallpaper scraps, and other printed materials. You can add other items, like string, yarn, and scraps of cloth. I also collect found items, such as bark, leaves, twigs, dried flowers, stones, and shells; you may want to add these to your box (see the "Basic Art Supplies" sidebar). You may want to look in an art store for interesting wrapping paper, origami paper, and colored papers or foils. Colored tissue paper is particularly interesting to work with because it is translucent, and when it is layered, undertones show through and create unusual effects.

Basic Art Supplies

The materials described in this chapter are helpful to have on hand for art making and the activities described in this book. However, if you want to assemble a basic supply list, the essential materials needed for the exercises in this book include the following:

- **White drawing paper**—a sketch pad or single sheets (18 × 24 inch paper is a good size because it can be cut into smaller pieces)
- **Pencils and erasers**
- **Felt markers**—fine and broad tipped, in at least the basic colors: red, orange, yellow, green, blue, purple, brown, and black

- **Oil pastels**—a box with at least twelve colors (twenty-four is better)
- **Chalk pastels**—a box with at least twelve colors (twenty-four is better)
- **Scissors**
- **White glue or rubber cement**
- **A roll of masking tape**
- **A box with assorted collage materials**—magazine pictures, colored paper, bits of cloth, string, yarn, found objects, glitter, sequins, and beads
- **Watercolors**—a box of twelve colors, in tubes, or a simple tray watercolor set
- **Tempera or acrylic paints**—the basic colors: red, orange, yellow, green, blue, purple, brown, black, and white
- **Watercolor paper**—a sketch pad or single sheets (18 × 24 inch paper is a good size because it can be cut into smaller pieces)
- **Palettes (on which to mix paint)**—a muffin tin, an aluminum pie plate, margarine-tub covers, or a plastic plate
- **A large jar or can (for water)**
- **Brushes**—synthetic: 1-inch flat, ½-inch flat, 1-inch round; watercolor: number 7 or number 8 round-hair brush
- **Self-hardening clay**—a variety of colors
- **A sketchbook (for visual journaling)**—9 × 12 inch paper
- **A notebook (for writing down responses to images)**

Recycled Materials

There are a variety of materials that you can obtain for free. If you look at what you throw into the trash each day, you will quickly start to see many materials that have possibilities for inclusion in art projects. Shopping bags, junk mail, gum wrappers, foil, wrapping paper, tea bag envelopes, string, and catalogs are some of the many recyclable materials useful in art making. Look at any containers, plastics, bottle caps, and other items that you might normally discard; put some of these items into a box and keep them handy for future use and inspiration.

Clay

Clay is malleable and allows you to explore texture and three dimensions. Potter's clay is the type of clay that artists use to make ceramic objects and sculptures. It is basically made from earth and water, is available at most art stores, and is inexpensive. Mexican clay is similar to potter's clay, but, unlike potter's clay, it is self-hardening and does not require a kiln (oven) to bake it. There are synthetic brands of self-hardening clay—for example, Model Magic—that are very easy to use and can be painted with acrylic paints. Plasticine and the familiar Play-Doh are two other forms of clay that come in a wide range of colors. Plasticine hardens but does not dry completely, so it can be reworked at a future time and used for other projects.

Experimenting with Materials

I generally ask people who have not used art materials for a long time simply to experiment with drawing tools, paints, and collage materials. This gives them an idea of how various materials feel and react and an initial idea of which materials they may like more than others. Learning about what different materials do and how they feel helps people enlarge their visual language and more easily develop imagery.

As an art therapist, I am also interested in seeing how people express themselves through different materials. Observing how a person uses materials gives me an idea of the materials a person seems to have a preference for or has a tendency to be more creative with. For example, some people are more expressive with paint, while others are inspired or stimulated by collage. While preferences and expression change over time, an important starting point is knowing with which materials you personally resonate and are comfortable. The following two experientials will help you find out more about materials and what they can do.

Experiential 1: Working with Drawing Materials

Materials: ten sheets of 9 × 12 inch white drawing paper and drawing materials (pencils, felt markers, oil pastels, and chalk pastels)

You are going to be working spontaneously, so make an agreement with yourself not to censor or judge anything you make during this exercise.

1. Have all the materials you need for this exercise ready and in front of you.
2. Working as quickly as you feel comfortable, use several types of pencils to make lines (straight, wavy, squiggly, and so on) across a sheet of paper. Try changing the pressure of your strokes and using the pencils to shade in areas between the lines. Don't worry about what your drawing looks like, and just doodle if you can't think of any lines to make. Move on to the next paper when your paper is filled with lines, and do at least one more page filled with lines and shading. Do at least two pages of pencil experiments.
3. Using felt-tip markers, repeat the exercise (Figure 5.1). See how many different kinds of lines and shapes you can make with the markers and how thick and thin markers respond. On another sheet of paper, repeat the exercise using only your favorite colors. Finally, on a third piece of paper, repeat the exercise using your least favorites.
4. Using oil pastels, repeat the exercise, working with all the colors you have in your set and experimenting with favorite and least favorite colors. Try mixing two or more colors on the paper and softening edges or lines with a tissue. Try creating a grid on one piece of paper and

quickly filling in each box with different shapes, lines, and images (Figure 5.2).

5. Using chalk pastels, repeat the exercise once more. Do at least two quick pages of experiments with the pastels, trying to make different lines by using the tips and the sides of the sticks. As with the pencil drawing, try shading in areas of the page with color. You can also experiment with blending two or more colors together on the paper, as in the oil-pastel experiment.

You may want to play music while doing this exercise and allow the music to carry your movements of the materials on paper.

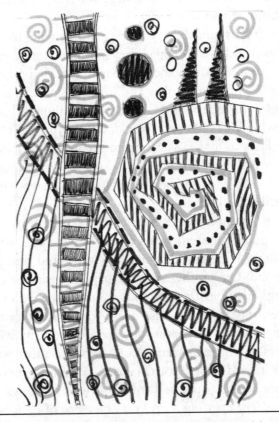

Figure 5.1 Experimenting with lines and shapes with drawing materials

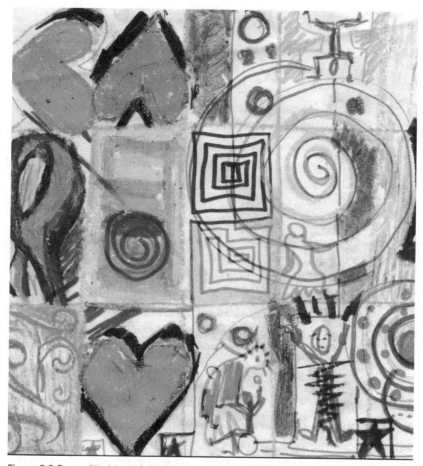

Figure 5.2 Boxes filled in with shapes and lines

Instrumental music with an energetic rhythm or percussion pieces are good choices.

Think about your color choices in steps 3 and 4, and list the reasons why you like some colors and not others. Look at the lines and shapes you made, and note which ones you like and dislike. Save these drawings, no matter how primitive they look. You may want to refer to them later, compare them to future pieces, or use portions of them for a collage or other work.

Experiential 2: Playing with Shapes

Materials: a soft lead pencil, colored pencils, and several sheets of white drawing paper

1. Working as quickly as you feel comfortable, use a soft lead pencil or colored pencils to make three or more of the following shapes on paper: square, circle, oval, rectangle, and triangle. Work spontaneously, trying to turn the paper around as you draw and overlap shapes if it feels right to you.
2. Use pencil to shade in areas between the lines. Again, don't worry about what your drawing looks like—just doodle and see what emerges.
3. Try a second experiment on a new piece of paper, using pencil to create a drawing with at least three overlapping shapes. Look at this drawing, turning it around and viewing it from several angles, and see if you can find a new shape in your drawing. Use pencil to shade or color in and around this shape, and add lines or other shapes to your drawing (Figure 5.3).

You can also try this exercise with other drawing materials, such as oil pastels and chalk pastels. The more times you experiment with this exercise, the more comfortable you will become with materials and your ability to create spontaneous images, the subject of Chapter 6. Developing and exploring your own personal visual vocabulary is central to experiencing art as therapy for self-discovery and satisfaction.

Experiential 3: Playing with Paint

Materials: watercolors, tempera or acrylic paints, brushes, three sheets of watercolor paper, and gesso (optional)

As in the experiments with drawing materials, you are going to be working spontaneously, so make an agreement with yourself not to censor or judge anything you make during this exercise. If you are working with tempera or acrylic paints, you may want to pre-

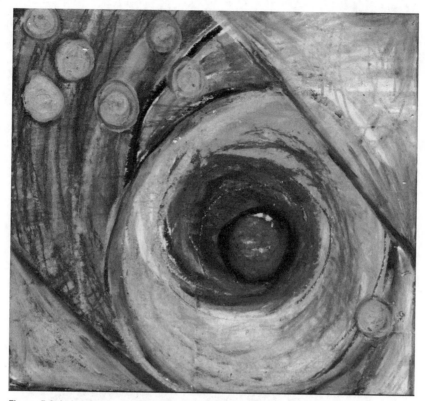

Figure 5.3 A drawing made from three overlapping shapes

pare the watercolor paper with a coat of gesso. This will take about an hour to dry, so do this well in advance. You can also paint with tempera or acrylic on any heavy cardboard, with or without gesso.

1. Set out your materials (paints and brushes), a large jar of water, and paper towels for cleaning brushes.
2. If you are using watercolors in tubes or acrylic paints, put a small amount of each color on a plastic or aluminum plate. An old Styrofoam egg carton is a good palette for tempera paints; put a little of each color into each compartment.
3. You will be using the three sheets of paper or painting surfaces to experiment with paint. Try any or all of the

following: use a large brush to coat the paper with water and try painting on a wet surface (this is called a wash); use each brush to see what kinds of lines you can make, turning them on their sides and using them to make thin and thick lines; try using paint without any water at all and "dry brush" lines and shapes with synthetic brushes; try mixing colors together on your palette and directly on the paper or painting surface; try using a facial tissue or a crumpled piece of paper to blot up wet paint or use cotton swabs or paper to make marks in wet paint (Figure 5.4).

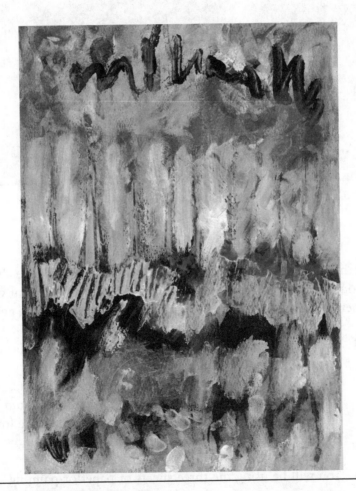

Figure 5.4 Playing with paint

Don't be afraid to invite some chaos into your picture—
try painting like a four-year-old child, discovering lines
and colors for the first time.

After you have completed three painting experiments, look at
them and jot down some of your responses to the colors, lines, and
shapes. Note how you felt about wet painting versus dry-brush
painting and how you like using materials such as tissue, crumpled
paper, or swabs to make marks in paint. Save these experiments; as
with the drawing experiments, you may want to compare them with
future paintings, use them to try out additional techniques, or create a collage or another project using them.

Experiential 4: Experimenting with Collage

Materials: magazines, large heavy white paper (9 × 12 inch or
larger), scissors, and a glue stick

Spend a few minutes quickly looking through the magazines.
Cut or tear out pictures and words that attract you. As with the previous exercises, don't think too much about what you are selecting
or how you will use them.

1. Set out your materials, laying out all the images and words
   so that you can see them.
2. Pick out images and words that catch your eye. Decide
   whether you want to cut or tear them further.
3. Arrange your images and words on the white paper. Once
   you have a placement you like, glue them on the paper
   (Figure 5.5).

When you have completed your collage, tack it up on a bulletin
board or wall. Write down some of your responses to this activity.
Think about how you used the images. Do they relate to each other
in some way? Did you choose to cut or tear certain images? If you
used words in your collage, how did you use them? Put your collage away and revisit it in a few days to see if you have any new
impressions about the images you selected. You may find that the
images and words you selected take on new meanings over time.

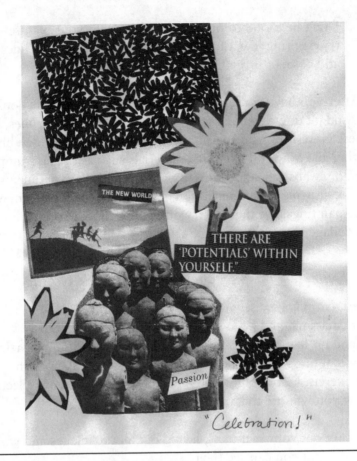

Figure 5.5 An example of a free-form collage

Experiential 5: Experimenting with Clay

Materials: potter's clay, plasticine, or Play-Doh; and an old rolling pin, combs, pencils, utensils, natural objects, and waxed paper

1. Set out your clay and your materials.
2. Try rolling out the clay between two sheets of waxed paper with the rolling pin. Use combs, pencils, utensils, and other items to make shapes or emboss the clay with lines, forms, and patterns.
3. Use a piece of clay to practice being in a state of play. Try different motions such as pressing, pulling, flattening, or

building without any preconceived notions about a product. Work with the clay spontaneously, and let yourself explore without rules or objectives.

4. Because clay is a tactile material, it engages the senses—sight, touch, sound, and smell. Try using clay to induce relaxation by holding a fistful of plasticine or potter's clay in your hands, closing your eyes, and letting go of stress in your body as described in the exercise in Chapter 4. Once you become aware of your breathing, begin to press your thumbs into the clay in rhythm with your breath. Let your breathing direct your fingers' movement into the clay for ten to fifteen minutes.

Keeping an Art Therapy Portfolio

Looking at one's work over time is part of the art therapy process. When people work with me on an individual basis, I suggest that they retain their work or that they leave it with me to store for them. This allows us to look at all the work at a future date and to review the images and content and see what changes have occurred. Many art therapists periodically review people's art expressions or, when therapy ends, use a session to review the work that has been done during past sessions.

Reviewing work helps people begin to value the images they make. Art therapists, like all helping professionals, respect their patients but also have great respect for the images that their patients create. This respect for people's creative abilities and self-expression through art is an essential part of the art therapy process. Encouraging people to keep their work in good condition and in a safe place conveys the sense that their images and their creative abilities are valuable.

If you try the exercises in this book, it is important that you keep your completed work and works in progress in one place, such as an artist portfolio or folder. Portfolios come in various sizes; I suggest that you buy one that is at least 24 × 32 inches to hold larger drawings, paintings, and other flat work. You may want to purchase a couple, one small and one large, for storing flat work of various sizes. They can be purchased at an art store or through art supply catalogs and vary a great deal in price. A simple brown folder with plastic handles is a good place to start.

If cost is a concern, you can also make a simple folder by using wide masking tape to tape together two large pieces of corrugated cardboard from large boxes. Refrigerator or large appliance boxes are good for this and are easy to obtain from stores. You can also purchase two pieces of a heavy type of cardboard called mat or museum board from an art supply store.

Visual Journals

In the next few chapters I will be talking about keeping various visual journals with specific themes, directions, or materials. These are simply sketchbooks or artists' journals in which you regularly draw, paint, or create collages. I often ask people in art therapy to keep a visual journal, usually as a form of homework between sessions. The process of keeping a visual journal helps you stay connected to image making, keep ideas flowing, and develop your visual language. In this way, it serves as a sort of transitional object—one that helps you see progress and growth achieved in therapy.

The idea of a journal usually connotes a diary or another place where one can express oneself privately with words. You may be familiar with *The Diary of a Young Girl* by Anne Frank, the young Jewish girl who wrote about her life in hiding during World War II. Other writers, such as Anaïs Nin and May Sarton, wrote about their lives in a similar manner.

Journal keeping, recognized for its psychological benefits, has been used in therapy for emotional expression and reparation. It has helped many people through difficult emotional periods, serious illness, or traumatic loss. It is also a creative process of self-expression and exploration of one's relationship to the world. A journal is a trusted confidant that helps us discover and express what is important in our lives. Art therapist Lucia Capacchione, who has promoted the use of creative journals for health and well-being, calls them "the art of finding yourself."

To begin keeping a visual journal, choose a sketchbook with paper that is appropriate for the media you plan to use. An all-purpose 11 × 14 inch sketchbook with a spiral binding is fine. There are more expensive bound sketchbooks and artists' journals that are good for pencil drawings, oil pastels, and felt-pen work. You can also bring loose paper to your local copy store, have it cut to any size you wish, and put a spiral binding on it. If you find you like to work on different sizes and types of papers, a loose-leaf visual journal may be more appropriate. You can keep your individual pieces in a folder or portfolio. Be sure to number and date them so you will know in what order you created them.

In addition to drawing and creating images in your journal, I personally feel it is important to write a response to the images you create. Chapter 10 describes ways in which art therapists approach working with people's art expressions. However, in initially keeping a visual journal, simply giving your image a title and writing several phrases or sentences about it is very helpful (Figure 5.6).

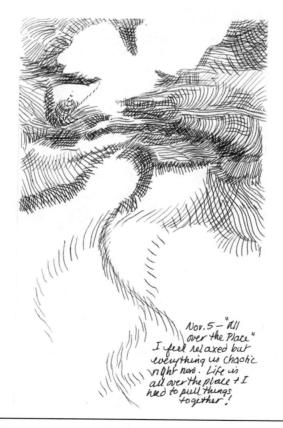

Figure 5.6 An example from a visual journal

Keeping a visual journal, like a written diary, takes commitment. I encourage people in art therapy to try to make an image each day, if possible, or at least several times between sessions. In the next few chapters, ideas for creating various visual journals are described. One of the best ways to start a visual journal is with spontaneous image making, the subject of the next chapter.

6

Spontaneous Art: Drawing Out Imagery

IN ART THERAPY, there are two kinds of approaches to art making: directive, which means the task has a specific theme or instructions, and nondirective, meaning there is no specific subject matter or particular way of doing the task. For example, if I say to you, "Draw a picture of your family," that is a directive approach because you are requested to make an image of something specific. However, if I say to you, "Draw a picture of whatever you like," that is a nondirective request. This way of working is sometimes called spontaneous art, free art, or free art expression, meaning there is no particular directive or theme given. Spontaneous art refers to drawings, paintings, or other art forms that are created without any preconceived notion of what one is going to make. Carla, whom I described in Chapter 1, was working in a nondirective way. She simply drew and painted what she felt, without any particular themes in mind. Carla intuitively used art to express herself freely and to create images from memories, feelings, and flashbacks to her childhood.

Both nondirective and directive approaches are valuable and are used at different points in art therapy. Art therapists often choose to be nondirective or directive, depending on the particular individual they are working with and the goals for therapy, assigning a particular art task in response to an individual's needs, interests, and preferences. In most situations, art therapists provide simple materials that are used to help people generate spontaneous art in the form of drawings, paintings, collages, or sculptures. While imagery that a person draws, paints, or expresses in any art form may be spontaneous, the therapist may provide a method or technique for creating spontaneous expressions; some of those methods and techniques are presented later in this chapter.

Art therapy has been strongly influenced by the idea of spontaneous art. You may recall the paintings and drawings collected by Hans Prinzhorn, described in Chapter 2. These art expressions by people with mental illness were made spontaneously; art therapy programs did not yet exist, and patients often had to rescue paper from the trash in order to find materials on which to express themselves. Their drive to make art is a powerful testament to the universal need to be creative and helped pave the way for the emergence of art therapy. As previously mentioned, the field of art therapy has also been influenced by early psychiatry, particularly psychoanalytic thought. One of the most common techniques used in psychoanalysis is free association, or saying whatever comes to mind, which is essentially a form of spontaneous expression. Freud is credited with developing this technique, which he employed to increase his understanding of how images, particularly those in dreams, were connected to his patients' lives. Jung developed a similar technique for working with patients and their images. Called active imagination, Jung's method involved observing the stream of images that spontaneously emerge in the mind. As a result of the influence of free association and active imagination, spontaneous art making became fundamental to the process of art therapy, because it encourages both uncensored symbolic communication and authentic expression.

There is now a clearer understanding of how the human brain creates images, whether through art making, imagination, or dreams. The field of neuroscience demonstrates that many parts of the brain are active during creative expression, depending on the type of artistic activity. For example, spontaneous movement of a brush across a canvas may predominantly involve areas of the brain related to motor skills. Making a drawing about a memory or an event, in contrast, requires information from many parts of the brain, including analytical and sequential operations, logic, and even abstraction. As more is learned about the brain, art making, and image formation, our current understanding of the theories of psychoanalysis, active imagination, and spontaneous expression will undoubtedly evolve.

Scribbles as Spontaneous Imagery

Many of the scribble techniques developed to help people create spontaneous imagery came from the work of twentieth-century visual artists who experimented with ways of creating art from the unconscious. Techniques such as automatic drawing and the painting method called psychic automatism were used to help the artist reach and express the unconscious mind through art. These methods involved creating images from the unconscious mind and expressing with paint or other materials in an unrestrained manner.

Margaret Naumburg, one of the first people to use the term *art therapy*, is known for her work with patients' spontaneous art expressions. Naumburg believed that spontaneous art expressions were an immediate and uncensored way of releasing unconscious conflicts in a visual form. These images, with the help of a therapist, could serve as a vehicle for self-understanding, especially when free association was used to explore them. Naumburg also observed that through this type of expression, many people found that they had undiscovered creative talent and were able to produce original and vivid art images even though they did not consider themselves to be artists.

Naumburg preferred chalk pastels and casein (poster paints) for spontaneous work, as she felt they were easy to use. She also taught people the scribble technique, a process that required large sheets of paper and either pastels or paint. Patients were instructed to relax their bodies in order to engage in drawing as freely as possible. They were then encouraged to draw without conscious planning by making continuous, flowing lines on the paper and by keeping the pastel or paint on the paper. When the scribble was complete, they were asked to look at the pattern of lines and to try to identify a design, shape, or object, person, animal, or landscape. The drawing could be turned in different directions in order to discover an image, which could then be developed, elaborated, or modified.

Naumburg was very clear that the images that emerged from using this technique were not meant to be used in diagnosis. She thought that it was a way to release spontaneous images from the unconscious and encourage free associations in therapy. However, some art therapists and psychologists have studied scribble drawings for characteristics that might reveal mental illness or emotional disorders. Several diagnostic activities used by art therapists include a scribble drawing as part of the tasks.

Florence Cane, an art educator and Naumburg's sister, also used spontaneous imagery, particularly the scribble technique, as a way to encourage creativity in children. She believed that emotions were an important source of both spontaneous imagery and creativity. Cane devised methods that included scribbling, movement, and sound to help children freely express themselves through art. Like Naumburg, Cane believed that spontaneous expression through art encouraged free association and revealed unconscious fantasies and thoughts.

Many other therapists have used what has come to be officially known as the scribble technique as a way to help people tap the unconscious mind and create spontaneous images. British pediatrician Donald Winnicott devised a similar technique called the squiggle game for use with children. The child and therapist alternately drew squiggly lines and would try to discover and complete a picture from each other's squiggle. The purpose was to allow the child to communicate problems or conflicts in a nonthreatening way through art expression, a natural language for children.

Using Scribbles to Create Spontaneous Imagery

Scribble techniques also have a connection to everyone's personal art history. We all began our expression as young artists through scribbles. Whether or not you made art as a teenager or an adult, you probably were spontaneously creative as a young child through scribbling lines on paper with a marker or pen, making shapes in the sandbox at the playground with your fingers and hands, or creating forms with a large paintbrush at an easel in preschool.

Children as young as eighteen months make their first marks on paper and eventually come to realize that they have control over the kinds of marks they make. By the age of two, most children are making drawings that psychologists call scribbles, and researchers have even identified a variety of specific types of scribbles that young children make. Most often, children begin making scribbles that look like dots and random lines on paper, progressing eventually to more controlled horizontal and circular lines. Since as young children we all began drawing scribbles, it is a natural place to begin in art therapy, especially for people who have not had much art experience or are unsure of where to start.

In the following sections, you will find some of the more popular exercises that art therapists use to help people release their flow of imagery onto paper and uncover their own personal symbols. Before starting any of these scribble exercises, you may want to use the relaxation exercise described in Chapter 4. Take a few minutes to get relaxed and let your mind become quiet. A good way to begin these exercises is to close your eyes, listen to relaxing music, or meditate. You may want to do these exercises to music; music that induces a dreamy, relaxed state is a good choice.

Scribbling with Your Eyes Closed

Materials: 18 × 24 inch white paper and chalk pastels

1. Place a sheet of white paper in front of you on a table or a wall. You may want to tape it to the tabletop or tack it to the wall so that it doesn't move around while you are scribbling.
2. Pick out a single chalk to use; the color does not matter, but you may want to pick a color other than yellow so that you can see the lines you will make. Place your chalk in the center of the paper, close your eyes, and begin to scribble around the paper. Don't worry if you go off the page; simply make a series of lines for about thirty seconds. (You may also want to try making a scribble with your chalk in the air before you transfer your lines to the paper.)

3. Open your eyes when you feel that your scribble is complete and look at the drawing. You are looking at the lines and shapes to see if you can find an image—a particular shape, figure, object, and so on. Turn the drawing around, looking at it from each side; if you made your scribble on a table, you may want to hang it on the wall and stand back to look at it.

4. Using any colors you wish, color in the image that you see. You can add any details to the image that you think are necessary or pleasing. Think of bringing that image into clearer focus by adding details, colors, and lines (Figure 6.1).

5. When you are finished, hang up your drawing and see if a title comes to mind.

There are two variations of this experiential that you may want to try. One is to do the activity with your eyes open. Some people are more comfortable with this way of creating a scribble; others find it less inhibiting and more freeing to create with their eyes closed. Choose whichever feels right for you.

The second variation is to use both hands to create a scribble. In this case, you can use more than one piece of chalk, holding one in each hand. With your eyes open, scribble on the paper with both hands at the same time. When you feel that the scribble is complete, look at it for an image. Because you used both hands to make the drawing, you may see mirror images of shapes, figures, or objects. Use chalks to outline, color, and add detail to your image.

Scribbling with Your Nondominant Hand

Another way to create spontaneous images is to draw with your nondominant hand (that is, the hand that you do not normally use for writing). Although many art therapists and others have experimented with drawing or creating with their nondominant hand, art therapist Lucia Capacchione is probably best known for her exploration of this technique. She refers to drawing in this way as the "healing power of your other hand."

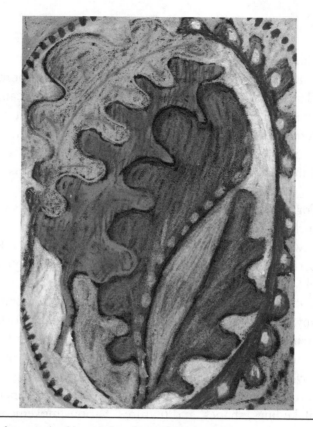

Figure 6.1 An example of images found in scribble drawing

You may want to use the materials listed in the previous exercise and try scribbling with your nondominant hand. When you complete your scribble, you can add details to make an image with either your nondominant or dominant hand; decide which feels comfortable for you. While Capacchione infers that using the nondominant hand may access parts of an individual's personality that are previously unknown to that person, I believe that working with the other hand can be freeing and helps one create uncensored, spontaneous images. Using your nondominant hand can be particularly helpful if you are feeling tight or restricted when you take up a chalk or pastel to draw.

Ink and String Scribbles

Making lines and designs with string dipped in ink or black tempera paint is another way of making scribbles and creating spontaneous images. The lines that are created with ink or black paint can be very elegant, textural, and stimulating to the eye and the imagination.

Materials: black ink (water-soluble ink is best, especially if you get it on your clothes) or black tempera paint, cotton string or yarn, 18 × 24 inch white paper, and chalk pastels or oil pastels

1. For this activity, you will need to work on a flat surface, such as a table or the floor. Be sure to work on top of newspapers or a table or floor covering, because ink can permanently stain surfaces. I also suggest that you wear old clothing or a smock in case of an accident.

2. Cut a piece of string about 18 inches long. You can use any type of string you have available, although cotton string is preferable because it soaks up ink better than synthetic fibers. Dip your string into black ink; you may have to do this a couple of times to get the string saturated with ink. Drag the string across the paper to make lines, shapes, and textures. Various movements will create very different lines and textures, so try moving the string in several ways; that is, twirl it in a circle, dot it, jab it, wiggle it, or slap it on the paper. The purpose is to fill the paper with lines until you feel that the composition is completed.

3. When you are satisfied with this ink scribble, go on to make two more; this will allow some time for the first one to dry.

4. Take the first ink scribble you did and turn it upside down or sideways, until you see an image, a shape, or a form that you like. As in the previous chalk scribble exercise, you may see something that looks like a particular object, face, person, animal, or landscape. Using chalk pastels or oil pastels, develop that image, adding whatever you think is pleasing or necessary to complete it.

Paint Blots

This experiential starts out with images that look similar to those used in the Rorschach test, which psychologists have used to evaluate personality. While you are not going to be taking an ink-blot test, you are going to make your own blots using paint on paper to create spontaneous designs.

Materials: three sheets of 18 × 24 inch white paper (you may want to cut this paper down to a smaller size or into a square if that seems appropriate), watercolors (tray or tubes; but if you use tubes, place a small amount of each color on a plastic palette or plate), a brush, a jar for water, and chalk pastels or oil pastels

1. Be prepared to work quickly during the first part of this activity. Take the paper and painting materials and place them on a flat, horizontal surface. Be sure to have a large jar of water on hand.
2. Dip a large watercolor brush in the water and then into one or more of the colors on your palette or in the tray of watercolors.
3. Do at least three of these spontaneous paintings; by the time you have finished the third painting, your first one should be completely dry.
4. Look at your first painting, turning it sideways and upside down as you did with the previous scribble exercises, until some image, shape, or form catches your eye. As in the chalk scribble exercise, you may see something that looks like a particular object, face, person, animal, or landscape. Using chalk pastels or oil pastels, develop that image, adding whatever you would like to complete it.
5. When you feel your first painting is finished, give it a title. Then go on and complete the other two paintings.

An example of a paint-blot piece is provided in Figure 6.2. Don't worry if your images are not symmetrical. While folding the paper in half often makes a mirror image and a symmetrical pattern, your drawing and embellishment of the shapes do not have to be bal-

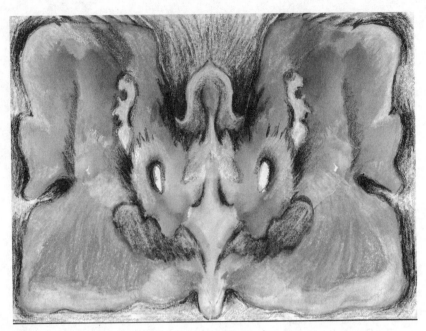

Figure 6.2 *Bird Mask*, an example of a paint-blot exercise

anced or the same on each side. Just go with what you see in the paint and use colors and lines to create an image in the shapes.

Working with Spontaneous Scribbles and Images

For many people, the process of freely working with materials to make scribbles and spontaneous images is creative, relaxing, and liberating. If you have taken a studio art class, it may feel very different to experience art making in this way, which involves simple techniques and no rules. If you consider yourself a nonartist, you may have been surprised by your ability to use your imagination to find images in your scribbles. Many beginning art experientials used by art therapists are designed to be accessible and successful experiences through which all individuals can create and communicate imagery.

While the process of making spontaneous imagery can be therapeutic, art therapists often help people go beyond the process to find meaning in their images. They use a variety of methods to do this, and some of these methods are the subject of the final chapter of this book. There are also a few ways to work with images on your own, without the benefit of a therapist.

While one drawing can have a significant meaning, as an art therapist I am more interested in a series of images made over time. After you've made several images, your drawings and content naturally start to develop, and your visual vocabulary begins to broaden. Because you may want to look back on spontaneous work after a few weeks, it is important that you date each drawing and give it a title after you complete it. Write a few phrases about it, such as your impressions of it or a description of the colors, lines, shapes, and content. If you are really ambitious, write a short story or free-form poem in response to it. If nothing comes to mind, hang your image on the wall or in a place where you can see it every day. After a few days, something will often pop into your head; record this description in writing, either on the back of the picture or in a notebook. Writing, in addition to art making, can be very therapeutic, as you will learn in the final chapters of this book. It also will help you to use the power of storytelling to give meaning to your images, connect thoughts and feelings, and help you discover personal symbols over a period of time.

I usually tell people who come to my practice that it may be helpful to have an intention (as described in Chapters 3 and 4) or a question they would like answered before they begin their scribble drawings. An intention or an unanswered question may set the stage for the mind to create an answer or message through the art image. While it may not work each and every time, you may be surprised at what emerges if you try it before you begin your work.

A Gallery of Spontaneous Imagery

It may be helpful to see examples of the variety of images created by people using some of the techniques already described. While these are but single glimpses of a number of images created in art therapy over months or years, they will give you an idea of how people in art therapy, some of whom consider themselves nonartists, used the scribble technique to create and develop spontaneous images.

Becca, a cancer survivor, came to art therapy to work on feelings of depression and to get help in coping with the chemotherapy treatments she was receiving to treat a recent recurrence of her ovarian cancer. She had first had cancer eight years before, and she'd had chemotherapy and radiation to treat it, but it had recurred two years after her initial diagnosis. Becca considered herself a nonartist and liked to try techniques that stimulated her imagination and creative thinking. She particularly enjoyed working with the ink scribble exercise both in art therapy sessions and at home between sessions.

One ink scribble she created in an art therapy session became a portrait of herself undergoing a particularly harsh course of life-saving chemotherapy (Figure 6.3). She described the image as "a woman with a turban caught in a spiral, spinning 'round and 'round." Becca often wore colorful turbans to our sessions to disguise her hair loss and to conceal the effects of her cancer treatments. While the drawing did not magically cure the depression about her cancer and the effects of powerful medical interventions, it allowed her a way to express feelings that were hard to convey to her family and friends and made it possible for us to talk about how she might be able to make changes in her life, given the impact of her cancer recurrence. Becca continued to use this method of making images throughout her chemotherapy, finding it centering and relaxing to work on her ink drawings while receiving treatments or at times when she felt hopeless, anxious, or sad.

A young woman, Tanya, who lived in Sarajevo during the siege in the early 1990s and had recently emigrated to the United States, found creating spontaneous imagery helpful in expressing her experiences of war and holocaust. Because she had witnessed sniper fire, destruction, and bombing throughout the city, Tanya experienced nightmares, sleep difficulties, and intrusive memories of the violence she had seen. In diagnostic terms, she was suffering from posttraumatic stress disorder, a group of symptoms that can result from exposure to severe trauma or crisis, particularly violence, warfare,

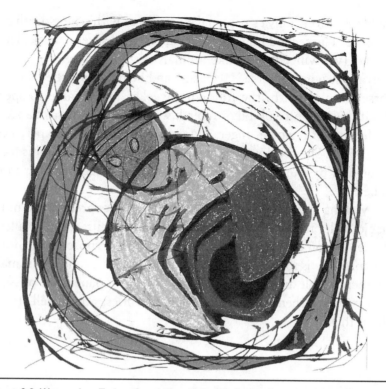

Figure 6.3 *Woman in a Turban Caught in a Spiral, Spinning Round and Round*, a spontaneous image found in a scribble by Becca
(Reprinted with permission of the artist)

or natural disasters. It is common for people who directly experience war, murder, death, or destruction to have some form of posttraumatic stress disorder and to retain powerful visual images of what they have seen in the form of dreams, flashbacks, or memories. Art making can be helpful in expressing this type of trauma and communicating the fear, anger, and grief that are associated with it.

Tanya created two particularly powerful images while working the ink scribble technique during a series of group art therapy workshops I was conducting. The first was an image of a skull entwined with black-stemmed flowers (Figure 6.4). While Tanya said very little about this drawing, the theme of death is obvious and understandable, given Tanya's personal experiences with seeing death and violence. The second image, which she created several weeks later, depicts two winged, horselike animals (Figure 6.5). According to Tanya, one winged horse is releasing and helping the other, smaller horse learn to fly. In the following weeks, Tanya came to speak about this image as a kind of rebirth within herself and a change in her feelings of remorse, anger, and depression about her experiences in Sarajevo. She continued to explore her feelings through this technique and by simply drawing and painting images as they came to her.

Making spontaneous images, like any art expression, is not a magic bullet for life's problems, and it cannot miraculously alleviate depression or long-standing trauma. The purpose of this form of expression is to communicate feelings, thoughts, and ideas, making them visible and tangible. Once they are on paper, it is possible to respond to them, to describe their qualities, and to tell stories about them.

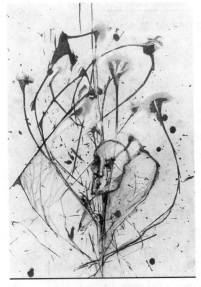

Figure 6.4 *Death Around Me*, a string and ink scribble drawing by Tanya
(Reprinted with permission of the artist)

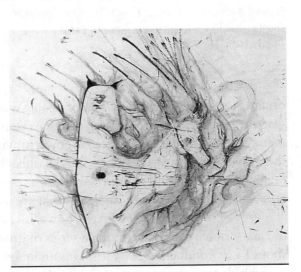

Figure 6.5 A rebirth image created by Tanya from a string and ink scribble
(Reprinted with permission of the artist)

Spontaneous Images Journal: Discovering Your Visual Vocabulary

Making images on a regular basis opens up many possibilities for understanding and expressing oneself. The idea of regularly making spontaneous images and recording responses to them was described by Margaret Naumburg, one of the founders of the field of art therapy. I often encourage people to keep a spontaneous images journal and to write responses to their creative work. By making images several times a week (or daily, if you enjoy the process), you may begin to see similarities in a theme, colors, or shapes. You also will naturally begin to develop your own visual vocabulary, by which I mean your own unique way of working with materials and your own images and symbols. Each time you work with spontaneous image making, you learn something new about color, line, and form, as well as how to manipulate the materials. And you increase your capacity to discover images in your scribble drawings, paint blots, or nondominant hand drawings.

Remember to give each image a title and write several phrases or sentences about it; you can record this on the back if it does not bleed through the paper, or use the following page of your journal to write your title and description. You may also want to keep a separate journal or notebook with your written responses. Although your images will be in chronological order, date each image every time you finish one. It is important to know when you make a journal entry, and it may be important to think about your image later on in relation to events in your life.

Choose a sketchbook with good quality paper, since you may be using a variety of materials to make spontaneous images. Some sketchbooks and drawing journals can take watercolor paint. If you think you may want to use paint in your spontaneous image journal, choose a type with paper that will accept watercolor without falling apart. If you find that you like to work on different sizes and types of paper, a loose-leaf visual journal may be more appropriate, or you can keep your works in a folder or portfolio like the one described in Chapter 5. Number and date them so that you will know in what order you created them.

To get started, use the simple scribble exercise described earlier in this chapter. Try to make a scribble a day in your sketchbook, look at it for images and shapes, and use drawing materials to develop a picture.

Mandalas: Making Spontaneous Images Within a Circle

The circle is a natural form to work with in art therapy because it has been an important visual throughout human history, extending to the origin of the universe. The spiral of the Milky Way, the orbiting of planets around the sun, and the movement of the moon across the sky echo the constant presence of circles. As children, we also discovered that we could use a crayon to make circular forms, meandering arcs, and curvilinear lines and spirals on paper. This is a universal stage of artistic development, which every normal child throughout the world experiences. It is also our first major leap in image making. When we scribble our first circular form with a felt-tip marker or pencil, it may be one of the earliest representations of the self.

Circular forms in art are often referred to as mandalas. In Sanskrit, the word *mandala* means "sacred circle," and Eastern cultures have used specific mandalas for visual meditation for many centuries. The Tibetan Buddhist Kalachakra, also known as the Wheel of Time, is probably one of the most famous mandalas and symbolically illustrates the entire structure of the universe. Mandalas are thought to be holograms of the cosmos as well as maps of individual consciousness. Mandalas and circular forms have been traditionally used in healing ceremonies in many cultures. For example, the Navajo people in the Southwest construct sand mandalas for the purpose of treatment of illness. These mandalas are large enough to contain the patient and are created in conjunction with purification rituals including sacred chants.

Jung is credited with introducing the concept of the mandala to Western thought. He noted that his patients often spontaneously created circle drawings, and he used the word *mandala* to describe them. He also had a profound personal experience with mandala images around the end of World War I, created his first mandala painting in 1916, and drew many more between 1918 and 1920. He described sketching in a notebook each morning a small circular drawing, a mandala, which he felt corresponded to his inner situation at the time. Jung believed that mandalas denoted a unification of opposites, served as expressions of the self, and represented one's total personality.

The mandala has been referred to as the reflection of one's psyche at the moment and a representation of a potential for change and transformation. Many believe that when a mandala image turns up spontaneously in dreams or art it is an indication of movement toward what Jung called "individuation," or self-actualization. Jung also thought that people created mandalas or dreamed mandala-like images as compensation for disorientation or traumatic experiences. He noted examples in his clinical work, such as children whose parents were divorcing and schizophrenics whose perceptions were disordered and confused. He believed the mandala image was encoded within all human beings and related to our need to resolve conflicts and dilemmas. In other words, when someone is confronted with integrating or synthesizing opposites, they may be drawn to mandala images in their dreams or spontaneous art.

Mandala Drawings and Personal Transformation

For many people who are struggling with emotional or physical problems, the mandala emerges spontaneously as a sign of change or transformation. It is often associated with a feeling of wholeness, growth, or the birth or emergence of something new. It can also signal a new understanding of the self.

Mandala images often appear in a person's expressive work when he or she is undergoing a dramatic change or overcoming a difficult personal situation. People who are experiencing serious illness or a life crisis may spontaneously create mandala images when they are physically or emotionally healing. The images can be quite striking, as in the following case of a depressed teenage girl I worked with at an outpatient clinic.

Joanne was a bright and attractive sixteen-year-old girl when I first met her in adolescent art therapy at an outpatient clinic at a university hospital. While she was intelligent and capable, she was not doing well in school and was having difficulties passing courses. She also missed a couple of days of school each week, saying that she felt too ill to attend. At an appointment with the school psychologist, Joanne brought a drawing she had made at home, depicting what she said was a "lady going down for the last time" (Figure 6.6). It was obvious to the school psychologist from the tone of the title and the contents of the drawing that Joanne was extremely depressed. She referred Joanne to the art therapy group because of her depression and concerns that Joanne was withdrawing from friends and teachers at school.

I met with Joanne weekly for several months, both in the art therapy group and in individual sessions. She was very interested in drawing and painting, and I encouraged her to begin to keep a "feelings" journal, in which, at least once each week, she was to make a drawing, visually describing how she felt. At first, she worked on drawings in her journal with my encouragement during her individual art ther-

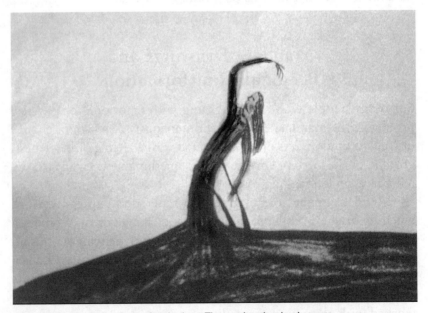

Figure 6.6 *Lady Going Down for the Last Time*, a drawing by Joanne
(Reprinted with permission of the artist)

apy sessions. Then she began to work at home, making several drawings each week between appointments.

Through her drawings, we both began to understand more about what was troubling her and causing her to feel depressed. Her first drawings were often abstract, a series of lines, colors, and shapes that were usually unconnected, chaotic, and disjointed. Joanne reflected these qualities in what she said about her life at that time. She felt lonely, aimless, and disconnected from others; she had problems with her schoolwork; and she had little interest in friendships. She did like art and felt that through art she could at least portray some of her confusing feelings in a way that words could not convey.

During the second month we met, her drawings began to change. While her previous images contained randomly placed shapes, the drawings now had a more distinct design and composition. She began a series of images she called "emerging stars," mandala-like pictures that seemed to echo her own first steps in recovering from her depression and withdrawal from friends. In one circular drawing, she began to identify her anger at her family, particularly her father, who had recently left her mother for another relationship (Figure 6.7). While Joanne had known about her father's abandon-

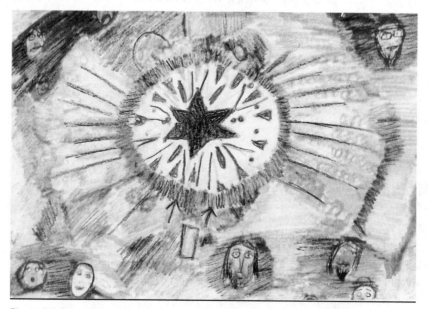

Figure 6.7 A mandala image by Joanne   *(Reprinted with permission of the artist)*

ment of her and her family, she initially felt that she could only express her feelings of anger and sadness through art rather than words. Her drawing journal was a place where she could communicate emotions and experiences too painful to say out loud or at home, where her mother refused to talk about the family situation.

Joanne used drawing to express herself for many months, and along with talking about her images with me and receiving help from the psychologist and friends, she was able to make significant progress with her depression. Her images continued to be mandala-like, and her drawings demonstrated a new lightness, space, and balance (Figures 6.8 and 6.9). Now as an adult, she continues to use art expression in her own therapy and as a psychologist with her own clients. While she did discover that she has a tendency toward depression because of her family history, Joanne maintains that art has been particularly important to her in expressing and containing her feelings.

I believe mandala forms emerged in Joanne's art not only because of recovery from depression but also because a circular form provides a degree of stability and structure for creating visual images. Working within a circle provides a visual experience of creating spontaneously within a structure and with a focus. In art therapy, I often ask people to work within circular forms or mandalas when they are feeling disoriented, scattered, anxious, or distressed.

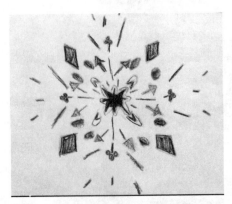

Figure 6.8 *Emerging Stars*, a mandala by Joanne as she recovered from depression
(Reprinted with permission of the artist)

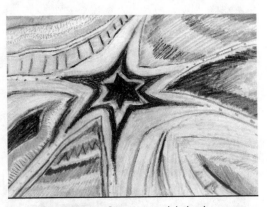

Figure 6.9 *Emerging Stars*, a mandala by Joanne as she recovered from depression
(Reprinted with permission of the artist)

Take, for example, my experience of working at a community drop-in center with homeless adolescents who had a variety of problems, including drug addiction, family problems, and lack of security. Creating mandalas seemed to have a calming effect on them, at least in the short term. Because of their problems, these "street kids" had difficulties focusing on any task for an extended period of time, and many were labeled hyperactive because of their limited attention spans. Because they could benefit from some structure, I asked them to draw within a circular format. The activity demonstrated how art making can channel our physical energies. For most, working within a circular form on paper provided a way to literally slow down and control or refocus often uncontrollable energies. While a mandala drawing will not magically reduce anxiety or troubling emotions, studies have shown that drawing within a circular format, as in Figure 6.10, can have calming physiological effects on the body in terms of heart rate and body temperature.

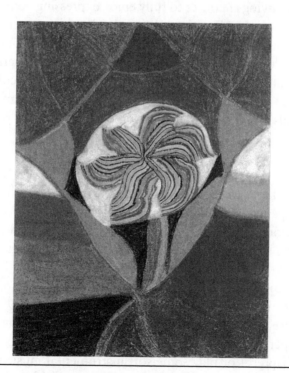

Figure 6.10 A mandala drawing by a fifteen-year-old girl

Making Mandalas

Making a mandala drawing simply means creating an image within a circular space. This can be done with any materials that you like: paint, oil pastels, chalk pastels, or colored pencils. However, since color is an important component of a mandala drawing, it is good to choose materials that offer a wide range of color choices.

While you can work within a circle of any size, some consider the size of the circle to be important. Art therapist Joan Kellogg, an authority on mandala drawings and symbols, suggests that 10½ to 11 inches in diameter is a good size circle for a mandala drawing. She bases this notion on the fact that this size is similar to the size of a human head. However, you may wish to use larger or smaller forms, depending on your own needs. Also, you may want to cut rectangular paper into squares for creating mandalas; the circle within a square was said by Jung to be a representation of the self.

I recommend using a forty-eight-color set of oil pastels for mandala drawings in order to fully enjoy expressing yourself within the "magic circle." Try drawing on both white paper and black paper in your mandala explorations. You may find yourself using different colors on the two different backgrounds and perhaps making different images. Also try other materials, such as colored pencils or chalk pastels, because different colors, textures, and qualities of materials affect the style and content of the images you create.

Mandala Drawings

Materials: 12 × 18 inch white paper and 12 × 18 inch black construction paper (you can cut both down to 12 × 12 inches if you want to work on square paper), oil pastels or colored chalks (try both; you may prefer one over the other, depending on how detailed you want to make your drawing), a round plate (about 10 inches in diameter) to trace or a compass, a pencil, and a ruler (optional for making straight lines)

Because making a mandala drawing can be a relaxing and meditative experience, you may want to start with the relaxation exercise in Chapter 4 or play some soft instrumental music to create a calm and relaxed mood.

1. On the sheet of white paper, use a pencil to trace the plate or use a compass to make a circle. Or you can draw the circle freehand if you wish.
2. Using the drawing materials you have selected, fill in the circle in any way you want, with colors, lines, and forms. You can start at the center or the edges of the circle; you may also want to divide up the space within the circle in some way. You may want to create a pattern or fill the space with a variety of shapes and colors. If you want to extend your image outside the circle's boundaries, feel free to do that, too. There is no right or wrong way to draw your mandala, so add to your drawing until you feel that it is complete.
3. When you have finished your drawing, put a dot on the top of your paper or an arrow on the back to mark the orientation (Figure 6.11).
4. Repeat the same process to create a mandala as described in steps 1, 2, and 3, but this time using the black paper.
5. Hang up your drawings, see if a title comes to mind, and write it on the front or back of the drawings. You may want to write a short description of the colors, shapes, patterns, or themes you see in your drawings, just as you did with the scribble and paint-blot exercises.

You will probably see a difference between your mandala drawn on white paper and the one on black paper. Colors appear quite different on a black background (Figure 6.12); you may have found yourself reaching for lighter colors, which show up more easily on a darker surface. If you try this again, you may want to purchase some oil pastels in gold, silver, or other luminescent colors, which show up well on black paper.

Keeping a Mandala Journal

Joanne, the depressed teenager I described earlier in this chapter, created circular drawings throughout her initial recovery from depression. Not everyone stays with mandala images for as long as she did.

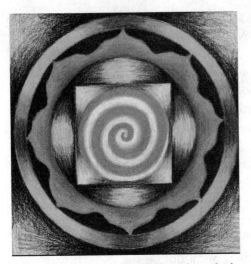

Figure 6.11 A mandala drawing from the author's mandala journal

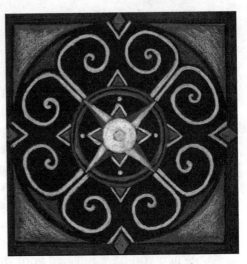

Figure 6.12 A mandala drawing on black background

You may find yourself drawing them spontaneously at certain times, or there may be days when you are less attracted to working within a circular format. While mandala drawings may reflect your inner self and feelings, you may choose to work with them regularly because the circle is a soothing form in which to work. Drawing or painting within a circle is containing, structured, and pleasing. I have personally found that creating spontaneous mandalas lessens anxiety, evokes inner focus, and creates a sense of calm.

Mandala drawing is one art process that is almost always useful to experience over an extended period of time. Keeping a mandala journal can be a particularly interesting experience because images often change and develop over time. There may be days or weeks when you find your images staying pretty much the same, and you may feel that you cannot go forward or away from the images that you previously created. But if you continue to draw mandalas on a regular basis, you will begin to see your drawings change in color, pattern, and content, as is true with other forms of spontaneous imagery.

You may want to select a sketchbook specifically for mandala drawing. Both rectangular and square sketchbooks are available;

you may want to use a square one for a mandala journal, because you will be creating a circular image. You can find various sizes of square sketchbooks at art or stationery stores, or you can have your local copier cut paper into the size you want and put a binding on it for you. Because it is hard to find a sketchbook with black paper, if you want to use black paper, you will probably have to get one made at a copy store. It is also rewarding to make mini-mandalas (Figure 6.13) on a series of square "sticky notes." Because these notes are so compact, you can carry them with you so you can make mandalas almost anywhere. I particularly like black notes because I can use colorful gel pens to create designs and images.

Decide what type of drawing materials you will be using before you select your mandala journal. For example, if you want to make mandalas with colored pencils, a small sketchbook either 6 or 8 inches square would be a good choice. Colored pencils will create more detailed lines and can be frustrating if you want to cover a large space quickly. If you are using oil pastels or chalk pastels, a larger sketchbook is appropriate to make drawings in; you will need a little more space because these materials cover a larger area with less effort.

Some therapists believe that specific symbols are found in mandalas. Since the mandala is thought to have universal significance and to represent internal states, many believe it reflects meaning through colors, patterns, and symbols. Joan Kellogg developed a system for understanding the thirteen types of mandalas, known as the Great Round of the Mandala. Specific mandala patterns, forms,

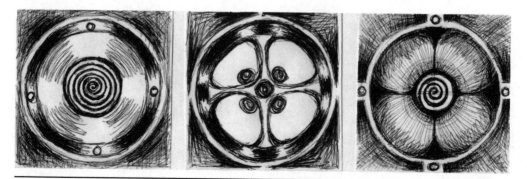

Figure 6.13 Mandalas on Post-it notes

and color use are thought to be indicative of development struggles, identity, personal styles of interacting with the world, and spiritual dimensions (see the resources section for more information).

For the purpose of keeping your mandala journal, work with the images as you did in the spontaneous images journal. Give each mandala a title based on your initial impressions of the drawing, and write the date on it for future reference. Look at the colors you have used, and make a note of predominant colors, listing your personal associations to each color (the topic of color will be more fully covered in Chapter 7). Describe the content of your mandala drawing. Jot down some adjectives, note the shapes or forms you used, and see if you associate any words, feelings, or memories with them.

If you take the time to keep a mandala journal and do some writing about each drawing, you may find that there are patterns and similarities in how you use color and shape and in the content and themes of your drawings. Don't worry if you don't immediately find associations and descriptions for your images; sometimes it takes a while. What's important is to experience the focus and centering derived from creating circle drawings. Of all the spontaneous art-making processes, mandala drawing is one of the most personally rewarding, soothing, and relaxing.

7

Using Art to Express Feelings: Drawing on Loss

Art serves as a helper in times of trouble.

RUDOLPH ARNHEIM, To the Rescue of Art

IN PSYCHOTHERAPY, IMPORTANCE is placed on awareness and expression of feelings, rather than hiding or avoiding them. An individual may be asked to talk about painful emotions in order to understand the source of conflicts and to begin integrating and ameliorating them. However, sometimes it is difficult or impossible to express feelings with words. Emotions, particularly those that result from trauma, crisis, or loss, are hard to articulate, and often words do not seem to completely convey their meaning. Because feelings are difficult to relate with words, many people push them inward, causing depression, confusion, anxiousness, hopelessness, or frustration.

Art making can be particularly beneficial in circumstances where overwhelming or complex emotions need to be expressed. The process of making art may help people confront emotions, overcome depression, integrate traumatic experiences, and find relief and resolution of grief and loss. Throughout history, visual art has been used to make sense of crisis, pain, and psychic upheaval. If you go to a museum, it is easy to see that human suffering has inspired some of our greatest artwork. Paintings, sculptures, and other art forms often depict traumatic feelings and experiences, artists' reflections and experiences of personal turmoil, or social upheaval. Van Gogh's swirling brushstrokes are thought to convey his inner emotional struggles, and Picasso's mural of Guernica, a Spanish town bombed during civil unrest, is a good example of how art is used to express and understand senseless acts of violence. Art making is a powerful means of making painful and frightening events concrete and releasing them.

Although there is a therapeutic benefit to expressing one's thoughts and feelings through art, one of the most impressive aspects of the art process is its potential to achieve or restore psychological equilibrium. Art therapy emerged from the idea that art can be used not only to alleviate or contain feelings of trauma, fear, or anxiety but also to repair, restore, and heal. Jung realized early in his work with patients and in his own personal explorations that art expression and images found in dreams could be helpful in recovering from trauma and emotional distress. He often drew, painted, or made objects and constructions at times of emotional turmoil or personal crisis. Jung recognized his expression as more than mere recreation and believed that it helped him find insight into his struggles. In *Memories, Dreams, Reflections*, Jung describes two important experiences that helped him overcome personal stress. He recalls a time when he was ten years old and found relief in making a simple wooden figure:

> I had in those days a yellow, varnished pencil case of the kind commonly used by primary school pupils, with a little lock and the customary ruler. At the end of the ruler I carved a little mannequin, about two inches long, with a frock coat, top hat, and shiny black boots. I colored him with black ink, sawed him off the ruler, and put him in the pencil case, where I made him a little bed. . . . This was all a great secret. Secretly I took the case to the forbidden attic at the top of the house . . . and hid it with great satisfaction on one of the beams under the roof. . . . I felt safe, and the tormenting sense of being at odds with myself was gone.

Jung also describes how he found relief from his traumatic break with Freud in 1913 through creating a structure with stones:

> I went on with the building game after noon meal every day, whenever the weather permitted. As soon as I was through eating, I began playing, and continued to do so

until the patients arrived; and if I was finished with my work early enough in the evening, I went back to building. In the course of this activity my thoughts clarified, and I was able to grasp the fantasies whose presence in myself I dimly felt.

Art therapy has been traditionally used to help people understand their emotions and recover from experiences of trauma, grief, and loss. As mentioned previously, art expressions have a long history as aids in understanding emotional problems, and drawings and paintings have been used in diagnosis of emotional disorders. However, the process of art making, rather than art's diagnostic value, has been particularly effective in helping people of all ages express overwhelming feelings and events.

Children's Images of Trauma

Joanne's story of self-exploration, recovery, and reparation through art described in Chapter 6 underscores art's powerful role in expressing feelings and healing people who've experienced traumatic events. In Joanne's case, her father's abandonment of her and her family precipitated her depression and withdrawal from school and friends. Although she was in crisis because of her experiences, art enabled her to express feelings about herself and her circumstances in a way that words could not. The process of drawing was soothing to Joanne at a time when she was particularly lonely, sad, and hopeless about life and her family situation.

Although people of all ages who have experienced emotional distress can benefit from art therapy, traumatized children in particular have taught me a great deal about how art can ameliorate emotional crisis. Most children, despite their experiences with painful events, still find joy and comfort in the act of creating art. It may be that through creation of art there is a natural experience of wholeness, and this, in and of itself, is emotionally healing. Based on research, we also now know that drawing appears to stimulate talking about one's experiences. For example, children who draw while talking about an emotionally laden event communicate more details about their experiences than those who only talk about it. They are also able to recall more details about the event and can convey that information to the therapist or counselor in a more organized fashion.

For children who have been abused or have witnessed violence, art is a way to express themselves when talking seems unsafe or when words are unavailable to describe their fears, anxieties, and other feelings. For many years, I have worked as an art therapist with children who have witnessed violence in their homes or have been themselves abused, and I have observed the impact of creative expression in their lives. Abused children, because of the personal violence and physical punishment they have been subject to, often feel uncomfortable talking, fearing retribution or punishment for sharing their experiences and feelings. Even very young children have the capacity to express their feelings about violence or abuse. During art therapy sessions, Paul, a four-year-old boy who was abused by his father, used drawing to communicate his feelings to me about his violent parent. Although he and his mother were staying at a community shelter and were safe from further abuse, Paul often used drawing to express ways he would control a "monster" who lived in their house and hurt himself and his mother (Figure 7.1). He would draw pictures and talk about a little boy who could overwhelm and disable the monster, thus saving himself and his mother from harm. Through drawing, he was able to express his anger at his abusive parent, and as his therapist, I was able to talk with him through his drawings about his fears of and anxieties about his violent father.

Paul, like many abused children, was able to use drawings to tell stories about his fantasies of rescuing himself and his mother. For other children who are abused, simply conveying feelings through art is an important experience, particularly when they feel that they cannot talk about them with a parent or friend. Being able to put on paper a sad or angry face or symbolically destroy or control a monster who represents an abusive parent can provide children with a way to express feelings that may not feel safe to speak out loud. In this sense, art serves as a buffer in acknowledging and expressing powerful feelings such as anger, depression, or fear. Carla's drawings, discussed earlier in the book, communicated her feelings about an extremely violent parent who abused her throughout her

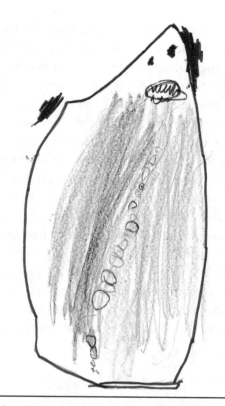

Figure 7.1 A drawing of a "monster" who hurts his mother and himself, by Paul, age four   *(Reprinted from* Understanding Children's Drawings © *1998 Cathy A. Malchiodi, Guilford Publications)*

childhood. Through her drawings, she expressed overwhelming emotions in a way that felt safe for her until she could confront and accept them. In therapy, Carla's images became a vehicle for conveying experiences and feelings and helped me to gradually guide her in understanding her past, overcoming her fears and anxieties, and resolving the trauma of having an abusive father.

In addition to helping abused children, art therapy has also been key to helping children deal with the emotional aftermath of natural disasters and catastrophic events. Children who have experienced tornadoes, hurricanes, fires, or earthquakes often feel a need to express traumatic memories and experiences through drawing the disaster for many weeks after the actual event. Children drew pictures portraying the destruction of the World Trade Center buildings for many months after the terrorist attacks of September 11, 2001.

Children who survived and were displaced in August 2005 by Hurricane Katrina in the Gulf region of the United States spontaneously used drawing and play to reenact their experiences. Tamara, an eight-year-old girl who was displaced from her home in New Orleans to another state, shared with me her recurring nightmares about her home and the hurricane. For the first several days that I worked with her at a shelter, Tamara repeatedly drew images of her experiences of huddling in the attic with her mother and brother while her home was being flooded with water (Figure 7.2). Through her drawings, she was able to express her fears of being in another storm and her family's loss of their possessions and their home. There is obviously a strong need to make images when one experiences trauma in any form and to repeat image making until relief is found. While Tamara needed many months of art therapy to emotionally recover from her traumatic experiences, art provided a means for her to communicate the sensory aspects of the hurricane and displacement as well a means of self-soothing and stress reduction.

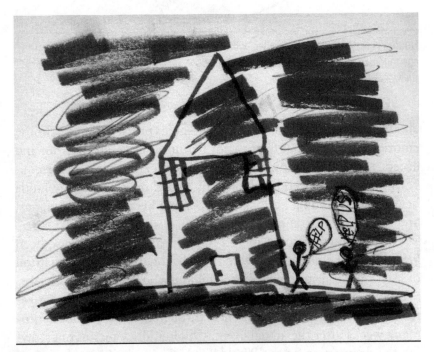

Figure 7.2 Tamara's drawing of Hurricane Katrina
(Reprinted with permission)

The power of art and the creative process in children's recovery from natural disaster and extremely stressful conditions were also clearly demonstrated following the December 2004 tsunami disaster in Southeast Asia. In his artwork, Fadhil, who lived in the region where the tsunami struck, portrayed injured survivors but also included rescuers, doctors, and nurses helping through providing medical intervention and supplies (Figure 7.3). Children like Fadhil who are able to communicate themes of rescue and assistance through their artwork often recover from the effects of trauma more quickly than children who cannot imagine getting help from

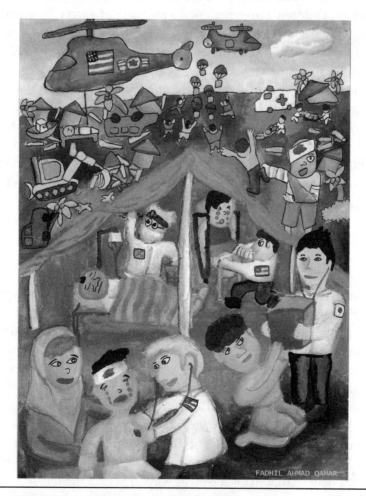

Figure 7.3 Fadhil's painting of the tsunami aftermath
(Reprinted with permission of the International Children's Art Foundation)

others. It is possible, however, because of the sensory and hands-on nature of art making, to help those children who are not as resilient as Fadhil to explore and imagine a safer and less traumatic world through drawing, painting, and other creative activities.

For children like Tamara and Fadhil, the process of art making is a way to gain symbolic control over terrifying circumstances and to establish an inner sense of security and safety in the wake of a catastrophic event. I regularly work with children who insist on carefully constructing their drawings, sometimes asking me for a ruler to make perfectly straight lines as if to exert control and structure through their art expression. Through drawing or other art activities, children can experience a measure of safety by virtue of being able to control the materials. They can also use creative activities to try to "fix" their homes, families, and situations—making representations that reflect the precariousness of whatever catastrophe they experienced and imagining ways to cope with the circumstances through art expression. For example, a child who has experienced an earthquake that destroyed part of the family's home may carefully draw a picture of the house and add elements to keep the building from coming apart. The act of drawing can provide an experience of control in response to fears of further destruction, providing children with a sense of self-empowerment.

Art as Emotional Healing

Adults as well as children have the capacity to use art to express complex and overwhelming emotions and to transform their emotions through art. Just as children who have experienced abuse or trauma naturally use art for expression and recovery, many adults have also come to discover the power of art to help them in recovery from their abuse or trauma, either on their own or while working with a therapist. Peter Levine, author of *Healing Trauma*, observes that adults working with traumatic memories must be able to access "body memories" of their traumas through the "felt sense" before they can begin to find emotional healing and well-being. I believe that art is a potent way to access the felt sense and the body's memories of trauma as well as transform overwhelming emotions that result from crisis. Elizabeth Layton is certainly one example of an individual who discovered that drawing enabled her to express her thoughts and feelings, particularly those related to depression and loss. Others have also found that making art, even years or decades after trauma has occurred, can begin the process of recovery and reparation. Jane Orleman is one such individual who has found art to be a way to self-understanding and emotional healing from severe trauma early in life.

Severe Childhood Trauma: Art Making in Healing Childhood Sexual Abuse

Artist Jane Orleman, who experienced sexual abuse as a child, has provided a rich legacy of how art can be healing and deepen one's understanding of trauma and help in the recovery from severe childhood abuse. Her therapist suggested that she begin painting from her own life experiences. She recalls how art she made during the time of her psychotherapy got her started on a journey of self-discovery:

> I have been a painter for twenty-five of my fifty-two years. In the mid-eighties, I began to paint less and less. By 1989, my production had diminished from an average of twenty paintings a year to only one. It was as though all of my vital energy and interest in life was draining from me. I filled the void with endless games of solitaire and science fiction.
>
> My mother died in 1989; this seemed to release me from my stupor. I began working with a clinical psychologist in 1990, with the hope of overcoming my creative block. As we discussed my early life, I came to realize that it still held a powerful grip on me. I found it very hard to talk about it out loud. I whispered a lot.
>
> I started to do one or two paintings a month. These images were inspired by subjects discussed in therapy sessions. I started a series of small paintings from the point of view of myself as a child. These child-view images have allowed me to say in paint what I have found so hard to say in words.

Orleman explores through therapy and her paintings her experiences of physical and sexual assault as a young child. She considers her paintings to be a dialogue with herself and believes that painting images has helped her accept memories of a traumatic childhood. She approaches her paintings with thoughts brought up in therapy and found that her art represented her unconscious telling her what she felt, thought, or remembered.

Guilt (Figure 7.4) is part of an ongoing series of more than two hundred paintings that Orleman has completed. This painting was one of the first images representing a narrative of her early life. Orleman adds:

> The secrets that I have kept until now have bound and contained me like this bottle of poison. The skull and crossbones mark the spot where all the painful emotions have been stored. I think it may be common to feel that one would never have been beaten or raped unless it was deserved.

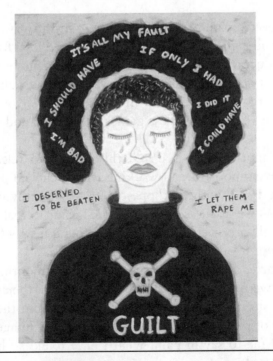

Figure 7.4 *Guilt*, a painting by Jane Orleman
(Reprinted with permission of the artist)

Orleman's art has helped her to make sense of powerful child-hood experiences and to process and ameliorate the effects of child-hood abuse. Through exhibits and a book on her art, her images now help others understand and confront their own traumatic experiences.

Art and Grief: Using Art to Find Meaning

Art has long been used to express not only trauma but also mourning, grief, and loss. The idea that art making can be helpful in processing a loss is certainly not new. Since early times, humans have used art to make important events such as death special through the creation of visual imagery, and art forms have been part of funeral ceremonies since Neanderthal times. It is clear that art somehow helps human beings cope with loss and that it is a universal human experience to express loss through symbols and to use images to relieve emotional distress.

The AIDS Memorial Quilt is an example of people's need to express loss and grief through images. In the late 1980s, when the AIDS crisis was at its height in San Francisco, activist Cleve Jones and others searched for a way to express the unending grief and loss they felt as loved ones and friends died. Jones and a small group of neighborhood residents gathered to express their experiences and to make what was the beginning of the AIDS Memorial Quilt. Although the initial project was a local event, word spread, and quilt panels from throughout the United States were sent to the San Francisco group. By the end of 1987, almost two thousand quilt panels were displayed on the Capitol Mall in Washington, D.C.

Since the original display, thousands of panels have been added. Together, they testify to people's natural inclination to make images to express loss and tragedy and the compelling power of images to commemorate those who have been lost. The AIDS Memorial Quilt comprises the work of mostly nonartists, people without professional art training or skills. It is an important example of how the desire to self-express through an art form is often heightened at times of mourning and how helpful creative expression can be during a time of grief or following a loss.

In times of grief, many have turned to creating visual memorials not only for emotional relief but also to remember, record, and immortalize someone who has died. When confronted with the loss of my cousin to AIDS, I found myself deeply drawn to the process of making a quilt panel. The creation of the panel took several months to complete, like the process of my own grieving. After working with various materials, I arrived at the idea of creating twelve squares containing photographs of my cousin and me, mementos, and remnants of cards and letters. This involved many hours of looking through old photo albums, collecting images, and talking to relatives to further illuminate the history of our relationship. I also spent a great deal of time writing in my journal and exploring my own feelings about death. After I had completed the squares, I carefully stitched them together and quilted the spaces around them (Figure 7.5).

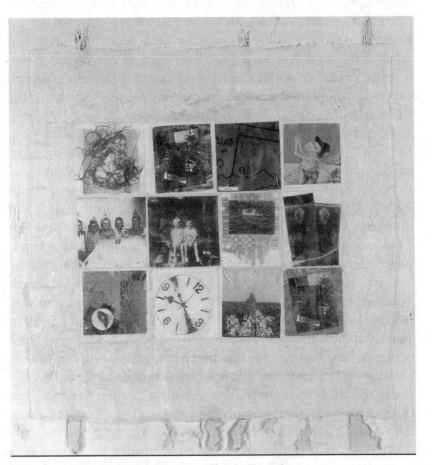

Figure 7.5 A quilt panel in remembrance of Ken, by the author

The quilt panel I created served not only as a memorial to my cousin but also as a container for memories, both pleasant and painful. It was a way to explore and understand my loss and commemorate a relationship important to my life and growth as an individual.

Art Therapy and Loss

Elisabeth Kübler-Ross, a psychiatrist who brought the process of bereavement into the mainstream, devoted a chapter of one of her books on death and dying to spontaneous drawings made at a time of significant loss or when facing one's own death. Because a person seems to spontaneously turn to art (as well as creative writing, poetry, and other art forms) when confronted with a significant loss, art therapy has become an important way to help people explore and express feelings associated with mourning.

Loss is a common and universal experience. Even under the best of circumstances, each of us faces losses at various points in our lives—perhaps the loss of a loved one, one's health, a job, or a home—leaving us depressed, empty, and confused. After a loss, some people become numb in order to avoid feeling pain, while others resign themselves to what has happened, burying feelings of distress and sadness. Because feelings are at the root of any loss, art therapy can be particularly useful, helping grieving individuals express their emotions and create a new view of themselves and of life after loss.

Art Therapy to Ameliorate Loss

Ben was a high-school senior when his mother died of cancer after being ill for many years. He had one younger brother and a father; his father was emotionally unavailable because of his own grief. Ben was referred to me for art therapy by his school counselor, who felt that he could benefit from making art and expressing his feelings through drawing and painting.

In our early sessions, Ben told me that he did not have much to say or to create in art. He made small, abstract line drawings, doodling with a pen in an absentminded manner. He was understandably numb from his mother's death. He also was exhausted from the many months of her illness, during which he had wondered daily if she would still be alive when he came home. Because his mother was very sick during the last year of her life, Ben told me he became "invisible," not wanting to cause any problems for his mother or the rest of his family. After all, his mother was suffering and did not have long to live. He wanted to be a good son and kept quietly to himself.

Although Ben created many paintings during several months of working with me, two in particular illustrate how art making allowed him to begin to understand his feelings and start his recovery from his mother's death. *Swinging Man* (Figure 7.6) is a self-image Ben created when he expressed an interest in painting. Ben did not take art classes in school, but he found that he was creative with paint and enjoyed working with watercolors during art therapy. He particularly liked this painting, which depicted him swing-

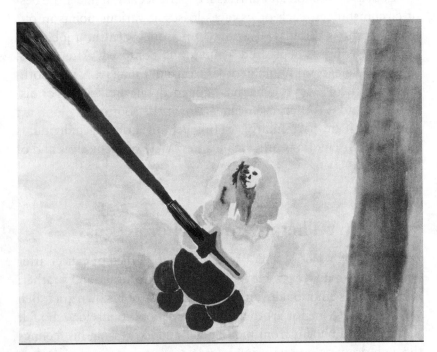

Figure 7.6 Ben's drawing of a swinging man
(Reprinted from Understanding Children's Drawings *© 1998 Cathy A. Malchiodi, Guilford Publications)*

ing on a rope, perhaps rappelling down a mountain or suspended from a bungee rope. Ben felt that swinging on a rope was an experience of freedom, but also the sense of being tied was similar to the feeling he had during the many months when he was in suspense over his mother's health.

Ben painted his self-portrait (Figure 7.7) toward the end of our sessions. He chose the shape of a mandala, a symbol of wholeness, and used many colors and shapes to paint a self-image within it. He described the painting as "half sad, half hopeful." In talking about

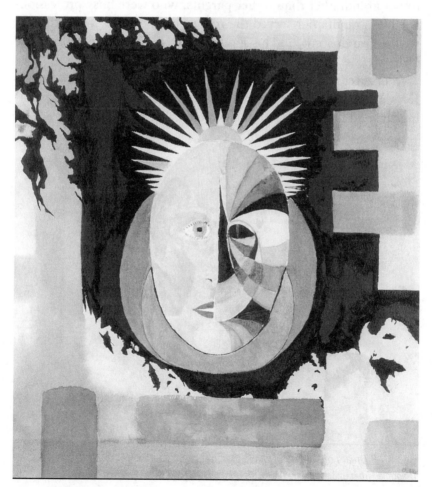

Figure 7.7 Ben's self-portrait
(Reprinted from Understanding Children's Drawings *© 1998 Cathy A. Malchiodi, Guilford Publications)*

this image, Ben reached the realization that part of his sadness stemmed from his anger at his mother. He recognized that he had spent many months thinking and wondering if his mother was OK while he was at school, at sports practice, or with friends. This wondering took up a large part of his life, and he felt cheated that he had missed so much during his high-school years because of his mother's illness.

Another teenager, Sarah, a gifted thirteen-year-old, went into a deep depression over the sudden death of her grandfather. She and her grandfather were very close; in fact, Sarah was actually closer to her grandfather than to her parents, who were busy professionals. Her grandfather served the role of both mother and father, as well as grandparent, and his sudden death created a great loss in the girl's life.

For several months, Sarah attended one of my art therapy groups for teenagers. One day she came to the session with a small painting she had done on notebook paper earlier that day (Figure 7.8).

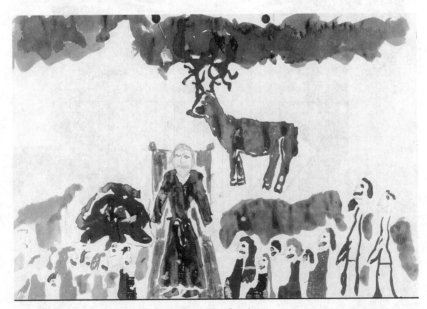

Figure 7.8 *Dream of My Dead Grandfather*, by Sarah
(Reprinted from Understanding Children's Drawings © *1998 Cathy A. Malchiodi, Guilford Publications)*

Sarah had depicted what she said was a powerful dream she had had the night before the session. In the dream, her grandfather appeared in a large chair surrounded by all his relatives, including children and grandchildren, with Sarah sitting on his right. In the dream, her grandfather gave everyone a blessing and told Sarah that he would be leaving her and he realized that she would be all right now. Sarah then saw a reindeer come down from the sky and lead her grandfather away. She was surprised by what she described as the "wonderful feeling of peace" this dream gave her, but she was also perplexed at the appearance of the reindeer that came to take her grandfather away. Despite the sense of confusion, she felt comforted by the image of the reindeer, and this experience enabled her to put aside much of her grief over the loss of her beloved grandparent.

The image of the reindeer in Sarah's dream could have been a way to self-soothe and resolve the crisis of her grandfather's death. However, for Sarah it was also a spiritual experience that helped her express how she perceived both death and life after death. Her simple painting poignantly shows her strong relationship with her grandfather and her feelings of resolution, and it is rich in metaphors that words cannot adequately describe.

For Ben, Sarah, and others who have experienced the death of a significant person, the act of making art is a way of remaking the self after a loss through exploring, expressing, and transforming feelings into visual images. In Ben's case, he had been preoccupied with his mother's health for several years, missing parts of his own life and spending his time worrying even while he was in school or with friends. Painting became a way not only to express grief but also to see himself in a new way after his mother's death and grieve for the time he had lost through his worry and preoccupation with her illness. Sarah used art expression to help her through her grief and to explore her own meaning of death and loss.

Art therapy has also been useful in helping people confront traumatic losses of monumental proportions. The use of art therapy with survivors of the bombing and destruction of the Oklahoma City Federal Building illustrates how art expression can help people recover and heal from traumatic loss of lives and process terrorism and violence in their community.

Art Therapy with a Community of Survivors: The Oklahoma City Bombing

The bombing of the Oklahoma City Federal Building, in April 1995, was one of the most devastating acts of terrorism in U.S. history. The bombing resulted in the loss of 169 lives and injury to more than 500 people. Survivors of the bombing and the families and friends of the deceased experienced multiple losses, of close friends, colleagues, and family members; many faced the prospect of attending dozens of funerals within a two-week span. As a result of experiencing a trauma of this magnitude, most suffered from what is commonly called post-traumatic stress disorder (PTSD). People with PTSD exhibit a variety of symptoms, but most have an inability to concentrate, a lack of enjoyment for previously enjoyed activities, a foreshortened sense of the future, physical complaints, and a fear of repeated trauma. Some have psychic numbness, or difficulty in expressing emotions, after the trauma. Others have frightening dreams or intrusive, repetitive memories of the original trauma.

Art therapy has successfully been used in the treatment of PTSD. It is thought to be particularly helpful in allowing trauma victims to communicate inner pain nonverbally and less directly. Victims of trauma, such as combat or violence, often have difficulty processing and verbally expressing emotions, a condition called alexithymia. Art expression can be particularly helpful with people whose trauma is so severe that words are not readily available to convey emotions that need to be expressed. PTSD is not limited to adults; the traumatized children mentioned earlier in this chapter often have PTSD because of their experiences.

Psychologist and art therapist John Goff Jones was asked to provide psychological intervention for more than 120 survivors and their families in the weeks following the tragedy. Jones used art therapy as his primary intervention to help these survivors express their grief. Because the bombing and aftermath were experienced differently by each person, Jones thought that art expression might be helpful in allowing these individuals to express the variety of posttraumatic effects, experiences, and memories each had after the bombing.

Jones presented his groups with specific tasks to help people express feelings, process grief and loss, build self-confidence, and reduce stress. An important part of the experience was mutual sharing, both through art expressions and communicating with each other in art therapy groups where both visual and verbal stories of the trauma could be supported. Participants were asked to explore feelings, to express anger and remorse, to compare themselves before and after the bombing, and to remember and commemorate those who died through simple drawing tasks and collage during the weeks that the groups met. They were also asked to keep journals to record feelings, both through images and words.

Jones felt art therapy was successful with the Oklahoma City bombing survivors for several reasons. The experience of the bombing was multidimensional. It was experienced not only on an emotional level but also on a perceptual level through images of destruction, injury, death, and loss witnessed at the bombing site and through weeks and months of continuous coverage on television and through other media. Art by its very nature is multidimensional, in that it allows expression of the emotional and perceptual world of the person. Because trauma often encompasses visual images and other senses through memories and dreams, art is a valuable means of expressing it. Jones also found that although many of the people he worked with had not found relief in talking about their experiences, they could quickly communicate aspects of their trauma through even the simplest drawings.

Like many professionals who work with severely traumatized clients, Jones knows that the therapist, too, is often overcome by patients' feelings and experiences. Therapists can experience secondary posttraumatic stress as a result of listening to stories or seeing pictures that express violence, pain, fear, and other overwhelming emotions. In response to his work with the survivors of the bombing, Jones used art making as a way to express and understand his own feelings of trauma, both from living in the community where the bombing took place and as a therapist responsible for treating numerous survivors. He had this to say about one of his images (Figure 7.9):

Overwhelmed. That seemed to be the dominant, overpowering feeling at the end of each long day spent entirely working with the survivors of the OKC bombing. Brave,

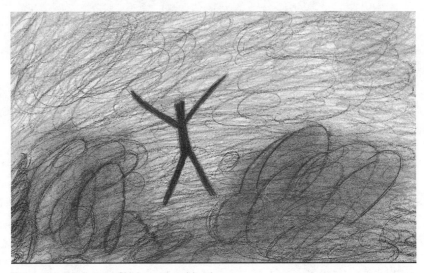

Figure 7.9 John's post-Oklahoma bombing image
(Reprinted with permission of the artist)

bright, devastated and completely overwhelmed by the sheer mass of loss, grief, confusion, and senselessness of this entire disaster, the survivors were desperately seeking relief, answers, and direction. How to do this with so many and in the face of unprecedented carnage against innocent civilians in the history of our nation? What to do, how to do it, how to even start? Unending questions, unending pain and grief and sorrow, and so much in need of relief.

More talking seemed only partly useful. Art therapy, a way to get some distance from the massive losses, to give vent to the anger, pain, sadness, confusion, proved to be most helpful. No quick cure, there was none. No quick answers, no immediate cessation of pain, but a glimmer of relief, a whisper of hope, and a hint of direction. Participating in the therapy exercises also kept the therapist partially grounded and enabled at least a modicum of orientation and direction for him. The images are still deeply ingrained in memory, and will forever be. Expressing these images, and the pain and loss they represented, allows these memories to be part of the therapist without overwhelming him at this point. Hard to ever portray the extent of loss, the dimensions of the loss, and the depth of loss these wonderful people and, to a great extent, the entire community experienced.

Feeling Journals: Exploring and Expressing Your Emotions

Jane Orleman uses painting as a form of visual narrative, expressing life experiences and memories through art. Her work is a visual journal of not only the traumatic events of her life but also her feelings about her experiences. These discoveries about herself made through art were helpful in therapy and allowed her own emotional reparation to begin.

Because you may not be an artist like Orleman, who was naturally drawn to working with images, you may have lost touch with art's natural power to express, explore, and ameliorate trauma and emotional distress. Unlike children, who naturally use art for self-expression, you may have forgotten that art making can be expressive of your inner world of feelings. To help people begin to explore feelings through art, I ask them to keep "feelings journals" as part of their art therapy. I have kept a feelings journal on and off for almost twenty-five years. In it I make drawings, paintings, and collages, some very spontaneous and simple and others more elaborate and detailed. I consistently find that these visual journals enable me to let feelings go and to get through difficult transitions in my life.

Art therapy emphasizes the importance of communicating feelings through visual form. In a typical art therapy session, people are commonly asked to express their feelings about themselves or others through art. Emotions are an important source for images and are a meaningful starting point in exploring oneself through art. Because we often keep feelings hidden from others, we sometimes lose our ability to communicate them. Expressing them through art is one way to begin to identify feelings that may be unrecognized or hidden. The very act of putting pencil to paper can begin to relax you, allow feelings to surface, and help you to put them into a context. Carla, whom I described earlier in this book, intuitively created a feelings journal many months before she came to me for art therapy. The traumatic feelings she was experiencing were frightening and at times unbearable; she used her journal not only to record her emotions but also to cope with them.

In beginning your feelings journal, choose a sketchbook that is appropriate for the drawing, painting, or collage materials you wish to use. Each time you sit down to make an image in your journal, ask yourself, "How do I feel today?" Try just drawing simple shapes and colors or cut out images from magazines to represent how you feel at the moment. Remember, no one will be judging your art. If drawing does not seem right, you can use collage, choosing colors, textures, and images that reflect how you feel or simply pictures you are attracted to. When you finish your drawing, put the date on it and give it a short title (for example, *Peaceful Feelings* or *The Way I Felt at Work Today When . . .*). Write something about your drawing on the back of it or on another piece of paper.

If you do this for a few weeks, lay out all your drawings, paintings, or collages by date and review your images, looking for similarities in color, shape, form, or content. Have your images evolved over time? Are there any regularly recurring emotions? How do you portray them? These are just a few of the questions you can ask yourself about the images in your feelings journal. Try to periodically write down some of the answers to these questions; this will help you discover patterns, forms, colors, and content that are part of your unique visual vocabulary for expressing feelings.

Examples from Feelings Journals

Many people I see in art therapy use feelings journals between sessions to express themselves or simply to relax and relieve stress and tension. A few examples of images from feelings journals are included here to stimulate your own creative work. While these are single glimpses of a number of images created in art therapy over long periods of time, they will give you some idea of how people use feelings journals to explore and understand their emotions.

Ellen, who had problems with anxiety and agoraphobia (fear of open spaces), used her feelings journal to record images of times when she felt panicked (Figure 7.10). She found this process particularly helpful in identifying situations and triggers for her panic attacks and used it to monitor her progress in reducing anxiety.

Paola, who came to art therapy because of relationship problems with her boyfriend, used her journal to explore feelings about their interactions (Figure 7.11). Her drawings were very helpful in conveying to me how she and her boyfriend communicated and what events precipitated conflicts in their relationship.

Kathleen used her journal to process feelings of grief after her separation and eventual divorce from her husband of nineteen years (Figure 7.12). While her art making did not magically cure her feelings of sadness, it was helpful to express her feelings when she felt particularly depressed or anxious. The drawings also were helpful in conveying to her therapist what she was feeling during periods of emotional crisis.

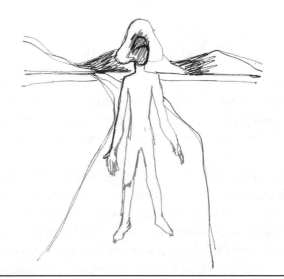

Figure 7.10 Ellen's feelings journal entry
(Reprinted with permission of the artist)

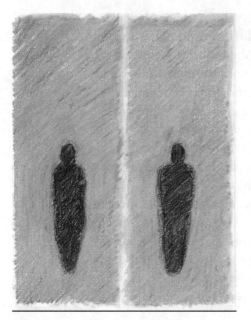

Figure 7.11 Paola's feelings journal entry
(Reprinted with permission of the artist)

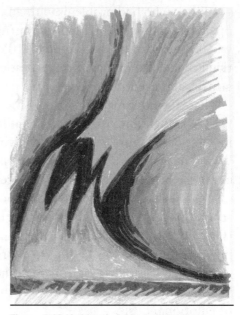

Figure 7.12 Kathleen's feelings journal entry
(Reprinted with permission of the artist)

Color and Emotions

There is no right or wrong way to express emotions through art. Each person expresses emotions in a different way, and we each have a personal visual language for expressing our emotional selves. Some people rely heavily on lines and shapes, while others find color more useful.

Although color may express our thoughts, perceptions, and physical sensations, we most often associate it with emotions. Noting and comparing the colors you use to express your feelings through images may help you to understand how color reflects your emotional self. When people begin to explore feelings through art, either spontaneously or through keeping a visual feelings journal, they often naturally wonder about color and how or if it relates to emotions. As you work with the exercises in this book, you will begin to see that you have preferences for certain colors or that your use of color changes over time. While colors often do relate to how you feel, it is difficult to place a certain meaning on the use of any one color in your art expressions.

You have probably heard such common phrases as "feeling blue," "red with rage," or "green with envy." We accumulate many of the meanings we have for colors through cultural influences. However, when looking at how you use color in your feelings journal, you may find that you have your own unique meanings for colors and color combinations.

The "Common Color Associations" sidebar describes some common color associations. It is intended to stimulate your thinking about color and its personal meaning to you. You will see from reading the sidebar that colors can have contradictory and even ambiguous meanings. For example, the color red is associated with both love and anger, two very different emotions. Many people choose blue as a favorite color and perceive it as calming and relaxing, but blue can also be associated with sadness or depression in other contexts.

This sidebar does not offer a definitive way to analyze your drawings or paintings in terms of color. It is provided to illustrate some of the more common associations that we have concerning color and to encourage you to consider how you see color in your images. Here are some questions you can ask yourself:

- How do you use color in your images to express emotion?
- Do certain colors have specific meanings for you?
- Does your family, religion, or ethnicity influence your associations to certain colors?
- Do certain colors remind you of a specific holiday or event?
- Are there colors that you wear for a specific occasion or situation?
- What colors have you used the most in your artworks? Do any colors dominate?
- Are there areas of heavy uses of color? Light uses of color?
- Do you like to use particular combinations, such as black and white; earthy, golden colors; pastels; deep, dark tones; colors found in nature?

Common Color Associations

- **Red**—birth, blood, fire, emotion, warmth, love, passion, wounds, anger, heat, life
- **Orange**—fire, harvest, warmth, energy, misfortune, alienation, assertiveness, power
- **Yellow**—sun, light, warmth, wisdom, intuition, hope, expectation, energy, riches, masculinity
- **Green**—earth, fertility, vegetation, nature, growth, cycles of renewal, envy, overprotectiveness, creativity
- **Blue**—sky, water, sea, heaven, spirituality, relaxation, cleansing, nourishing, calm, loyalty
- **Violet/purple**—royalty, spirituality, wealth, authority, death, resurrection, imagination, attention, excitement, paranoia, persecution
- **Black**—darkness, emptiness, mystery, beginning, womb, unconsciousness, death, depression, loss
- **Brown**—fertility, soil, sorrow, roots, excrement, dirt, worthlessness, new beginnings
- **White**—light, virginity, purity, moon, spirituality, creation, timelessness, dreamlike, generativity, resurrection, clarity, loss, synthesis, enlightenment

As you work with color, your preferences will change. For example, oil pastels will naturally lead you to experiment with blending colors. Try creating images using limited color ranges, such as cool colors (blues, blue-greens, lavender); warm colors (reds, oranges, yellows); or gray tones, black, and white. Or try making a drawing or painting with colors you would not usually use. As you experiment with new materials and color combinations, your feelings, meanings, and preferences for color will evolve.

Using Imagery to Create Emotional Safety

While expressing feelings is helpful, sometimes it is more important to use images to self-soothe and create positive sensations. I try to help people who are depressed, anxious, or in crisis to use art making as a way to take care of themselves, as well as to communicate trauma and loss.

Self-Soothing Image Book

Materials: at least ten sheets of 8½ × 11 inch white paper or any other colored paper of a similar size (you will be binding pages to form a book), magazines, colored paper, collage materials, scissors, and glue

1. Make a list of sensory experiences that are pleasant for you. Think about any of the following: environments or nature; sounds or music; tastes or scents; tactile sensations or textures; or a particular experience or event that made you feel happy, content, or peaceful.
2. Look through magazines and other collage materials for examples of images that could represent the pleasant and soothing sensory experiences you listed. Cut out as many images as you wish.
3. Create pages for these images by gluing them to paper. You can arrange them in a composition or categorize them by type (for example, outdoors, textures, and animals).
4. Collate the pages (punch holes to put them in a binder or take them to the local copier and have a spiral binding put on), and complete a personal cover for the book.
5. After you have completed the project, jot down some notes to describe your general thoughts and feelings while you were selecting materials for the book. Which sensory images did you favor over others? Why?
6. Look through the book and select an image or a page that is particularly pleasant or soothing. Take a minute to focus on it and enter into the sensory aspects of the picture. What do you experience when looking at the picture?
7. Feel free to add to the book whenever you find additional images you would like to include. If you use a spiral binding or school binder, it will be easy for you to add to the book at any time.

This exercise is similar to the one in Chapter 3 in which you identified images and objects that give you pleasure. The self-soothing image book is another place to keep such images (or colors, textures, and forms). A cancer patient used this exercise to develop a book of images to take to the hospital and look through while she received chemotherapy treatment. Looking at her images helped her to forget about the unpleasant effects of the treatment and to focus on her own recovery.

Another variation of this exercise is to arrange your collection of images on a large piece of cardboard or mat board and glue them in place. You might want to add a simple frame or a piece of Plexiglas and hang the collage where you can see it on a regular basis.

Creating a Safe Place

This is a popular directive used by therapists to help people who are in distress. The idea is first to create an image of safety to help relieve tension and second to discover mental images that enhance one's sense of security.

Materials: 18 × 24 inch white drawing paper and oil pastels or colored pencils

1. Start with the relaxation exercise described in Chapter 4. When you feel relaxed, think of all the places, real and imaginary, that have felt safe to you during your life. (If you can't think of a specific one, try to imagine one.)
2. Make a list of all the characteristics of your safe place (for example, things that are comfortable, such as pillows and furniture; things that are familiar; and things that you enjoy having around you).
3. Use the art materials to draw your safe place; you can make a simple diagram or an elaborate illustration. Add any features that will enhance the safety of the place or make it more comfortable.
4. Look at your image, and describe the significance and purpose of each characteristic or feature you included. Imagine yourself standing in this safe place. What would you see to the left and right of you, in front of you, and above and below you?

5. Look at your image, and consider under what circumstances your safe place would be most helpful to you. Note these.
6. Develop a picture in your mind of your safe place, and practice visualizing it during the next few days. What does it feel like to visit this place in your imagination?

Feeling Maps

This exercise is based on one that was used by John Goff Jones in his work with the Oklahoma City bombing survivors to explore and record feelings.

Materials: large white paper and colored pencils or felt markers

1. You are going to represent the following six feelings: anger, joy, sadness, fear, love of others, and love of self. Use a different color to represent each of the feelings. Try to imagine what each emotion looks like in terms of size and shape. Try not to use stick figures or happy-face characters to represent these feelings.
2. When you have completed all the images, consider whether any are connected to each other. How do your images relate to each other? Do any have common shapes or lines? How do they compare in size? Which one did you spend the most time on?

Painting Your Feelings

Because paint is one of the more fluid materials with which to work, it is especially conducive to conveying emotion.

Although there is no magic formula for painting your troubling emotions and finding relief or well-being, spontaneous painting may help you to explore and express your feelings. Try doing a series of small paintings of feelings. Prepare a series of surfaces, such as watercolor paper, cardboard, or mat board with gesso. An 11 × 14 inch surface is a good size to start. Using acrylic or tempera paints, choose colors that represent your mood or simply paint spontaneously, as described in the previous chapter.

In *Art as Medicine*, art therapist Shaun McNiff has some help-ful advice for beginning painters who are interested in the healing powers of art and self-expression:

> Just paint. Begin to move with the brush in different ways. Watch what comes. If you paint, it will come. Nothing will happen unless you begin to paint, in your own way. Start painting as though you are dancing with your whole body, and not just using your fingers and your wrist. Use your arms with the force of the body behind them. Look at the shapes that appear, and think about what you can do with them.
>
> Relax and find your own way of making images with paint. If you feel constrained or tense, try painting with your nondominant hand, or use the ink scribble technique to create lines and forms, filling them in with color or adding details with paint to create images.

Try painting merely for the joy of working with colors. Writer and amateur painter Henry Miller once remarked, "Paint as you like and die happy." Art therapy is about making art as you like, without concern for it being judged. It is about enjoying the pro-cess of working with colors, forms, textures, and images and tak-ing pleasure from self-expression. If you like working outdoors, you might try painting a landscape. But instead of worrying about being realistic and copying what you see, try painting from what is inside you. Try using colors that represent how you feel about trees, water, earth, and sky, instead of trying to duplicate colors in nature. Per-haps the sky feels warm and sultry to you; think about what color represents that feeling and what lines, forms, or shapes convey that idea. Try touching the things you see around you and painting the way their textures make you feel. Or, as McNiff suggests, paint from movement in your body rather than your fingers. Perhaps your body feels tightly knotted into a ball or stretched in all directions. Think about how you feel and how that could be expressed in lines or gestures across the surface, and see what develops.

A Final Note

While the exercises presented in this chapter can be helpful for you in working through emotional problems, there are limits to what they can do. If you have serious emotional problems or have had traumatic experiences, you may also need the help of a professional. Art making can go a long way in transforming emotional pain, ameliorating trauma, and helping to make sense of loss, but sometimes you need to deepen your understanding through work with a therapist.

8

Art Making and Illness: Drawing a Picture of Health

I wish all physicians would add a box of crayons to their diagnostic and therapeutic tools.

BERNIE SIEGEL, M.D., *PEACE, LOVE, AND HEALING*

ONE OF THE first uses of art therapy involved the treatment of physical illness. Adrian Hill, the founder of art therapy in Great Britain, used the term *art therapy* in his early writings to describe the impact of his painting on his recovery from tuberculosis. Hill went on to write two books on his experiences: *Art Versus Illness* and *Painting Out Illness*. Eventually, Hill brought art-making experiences to other patients with physical illnesses, setting the stage for the use of art therapy for people with medical conditions and disabilities.

The use of art therapy for psychological and somatic aspects of physical illness has grown for several reasons. First, increased interest in alternative medicine has led many people to seek out therapies that complement their medical treatment. Art therapists and medical professionals have learned that art can convey powerful messages, both conscious and unconscious, about our bodies as well as our minds. Also, the creative process of making images is an effective therapy for those who are confronting serious illness. It helps individuals cope with pain and other debilitating symptoms to identify feelings and physical symptoms and to become active participants in their medical care.

Images as Messengers of Health and Illness

The belief that dream images can foretell physical illness dates back to early Greek civilization. Hippocrates, a Greek physician and the father of medicine, noted that dreams could confirm one's physical condition; he believed that vivid images of the sun, moon, and heavens, trees thriving and in bloom, and rivers flowing were all signs of excellent health. Galen, an early physician who practiced during the second century A.D., also used the images in his own dreams and those of his patients to prescribe remedies and treatments and believed dreams were a diagnostic tool.

A dream image that predicts physical illness is called a prodrome, meaning an early symptom indicating the onset of a disease. Dreams have also been associated with physical recovery, spontaneous healing, and health remedies. Jung was interested in the possibility that dreams provided intuitive information on one's physical condition, which could lead to appropriate treatment. He was once asked to interpret the following description of a patient's dream without having any other information:

> Someone beside me kept asking me something about oiling some machinery. Milk was suggested as the best lubricant. Apparently I thought that oozy slime was preferable. Then, a pond was drained and amid the slime there were two extinct animals. One was a minute mastodon. I forgot what the other one was.

From the patient's dream, Jung correctly determined that the patient had a blockage of cerebrospinal fluid caused by a tumor or similar problem. He made this diagnosis from the images in the dream and his extensive knowledge of their symbolic meanings. While Jung's reasoning for this diagnosis may be hard to believe, it is easy to understand from the patient's description that the dream described a malfunction of some sort (in this case, a machine in need of a lubricant). This indicated to Jung that there might be a problem somewhere in the body, and other aspects of the dream suggested the idea of a blockage or tumor.

Jung's beliefs have led others to explore the use of dreams to diagnose illnesses. Dreams of people with tuberculosis have revealed images of suffocation, and people with ulcers have dreamed about holes in their stomachs. In both groups, the patients had dreams relating to their illnesses well before they were diagnosed. Dream images have also been studied in patients with heart disease, lung conditions, malignancies, and other severe illnesses, and certain dream images were found to be predictive of the course of patients' conditions. For example, men whose dreams contain themes of death or dying have been found to be more likely to die or to suffer a recurrence of their illness.

Dreams are not the only source of images that reflect or reveal physical health or illness. Drawings and other art expressions also can express symptoms, the course of illness, and critical changes in health status. Bernie Siegel, a physician who is well known for his work with cancer patients, observes that drawings can tell a great deal about the patient's condition. Recent studies indicate that children can communicate headache pain more accurately through drawings than with words and that their drawings are helpful to doctors in understanding and treating their headache pain.

Adults and children frequently express physical illness in art therapy both consciously and unconsciously. One little girl with whom I worked in an art therapy group for children from abusive homes unconsciously expressed in her drawings a recurrent stomach pain she was experiencing. Although she was in a great deal of pain, she did not talk about her symptoms and generally seemed calm and happy. However, to my puzzlement, she consistently drew or painted images with a black area in them (Figures 8.1 and 8.2). As her therapist, I asked her about the dark colors she used, but she would smile and say nothing, as if to reassure me that she was all right. Yet the repetition of dark colors in her drawings caused me some concern, and I wondered if they might represent some type of pain. Although I was certain that she had not been physically abused, I did know that she had witnessed the repeated physical abuse of her mother by her alcoholic father.

After the girl was given a physical examination by a doctor, I was surprised to learn that she had a duodenal ulcer, a very painful condition generally found in middle-aged adults. It seemed that the girl, in an effort to submerge her emotional distress, had finally expressed it as a somatic condition in the form of a very painful stomach ulcer. Children may use the colors black or red to express physical pain in their art expressions. This little girl used drawings as a way to communicate her illness and pain, feeling that she would be troubling her already emotionally distressed family if she openly complained about her stomach pain. She felt compelled to express what was otherwise unspeakable physical pain through the language of art.

This example does not mean that every use of black or a dark color in a drawing or painting is a sign of pain or illness. Both children and adults use colors to represent many feelings and experiences, and it is therefore impossible to say with certainty that specific colors, shapes, or content mean that there is illness or physical distress. However, it is well documented that certain images, forms, and colors may communicate information about illness. Susan Bach, a psychotherapist and researcher who worked for several decades with terminally ill children, noted that certain signs in their drawings fore-

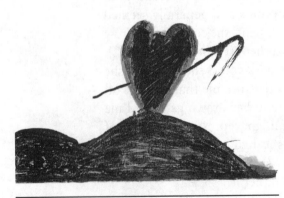

Figure 8.1 A drawing of a heart with a black center, by an eight-year-old girl
(Reprinted from Breaking the Silence: Art Therapy with Children from Violent Homes *© 1997 Cathy A. Malchiodi, Brunner-Routledge)*

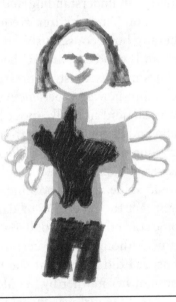

Figure 8.2 A self-portrait with a black interior, by an eight-year-old girl
(Reprinted from Breaking the Silence: Art Therapy with Children from Violent Homes *© 1997 Cathy A. Malchiodi, Brunner-Routledge)*

cast illness and recovery. These signs can include colors, placement of objects, or symbolic representations. Bach also observed that dying children are often aware of their impending death even before medical personnel or family and express their awareness through specific symbols in their spontaneous drawings. Bach's work underscores not only the idea that art images can express the somatic but also that body, mind, and spirit are inevitably intertwined.

Joan Kellogg, the authority on mandala drawings mentioned in Chapter 6, also has noted the relationship between color and physical health. Kellogg observed that in some mandala drawings, certain colors can indicate conditions such as inflammation, pain, nausea, stomach illnesses, or breathing difficulties. The use of color in images is strongly related to not only emotions but also physical sensations.

The Healing Powers of Art Making

The process of art making is recognized as being important to physical healing, whether in the form of recovery or rehabilitation, learning to cope with illness or symptoms, or finding meaning for the experience of serious or life-threatening illness. The arts in health care movement, described earlier in this book, emphasizes the use of all the arts in recovery from illness or medical procedures. Medicine has also learned that the ability to express oneself through art, music, movement, or writing enhances perceptions of well-being. The sense of well-being is increased even in people who are disabled or have chronic illness, underscoring art's ability to help individuals transcend and even transform their sense of self in the face of disease or physical discomfort.

Oliver Sacks, a well-known British neurologist and author, describes the quality of awakening that the arts provide to physically ill or disabled individuals:

> Awakening, basically, is a reversal . . . the patient ceases to feel the presence of illness and the absence of the world, and comes to feel the absence of his illness and the full presence of the world.

During art making, people often shift away from the presence of illness in their lives. They momentarily forget that they are sick or disabled and awaken to experiences other than illness. Also, as many patients say in their conversations with me on the value of the art process, art making is an experience that provides a type of transcendence. Patients observe that they can often rise above illness, overcome pain, and get past fears and anxieties while engaged in art making. This quality of transcendence may be one of art making's most potent therapeutic aspects.

Art making may also provide an experience of normalcy, if only for the time one is engaged in creative activity. In addition to shifting attention away from illness, art making can be a positive distraction for people experiencing pain or debilitating symptoms. Arthritis patients and others who have pain often report that they have reduced perceptions of pain during art making.

Finally, a person who is ill often loses a sense of control of his or her body as well as a sense of autonomy. People who are hospitalized lose control of time because they live their lives on the hospital's schedule. Art therapy can help people with physical illness regain some measure of control in their lives by providing the freedom to select materials, style, and subject matter; to play freely with colors, lines, forms, and textures; and to choose to create what they want to create.

Healing Through Art

Many artists have used art to express their own struggles with illness, disability, or pain. Frida Kahlo, a Mexican surrealist painter and wife of the painter Diego Rivera, painted many self-portraits that explored and expressed her struggles with lifelong health problems. Kahlo had polio as a child and suffered from a congenital condition of the spine that caused her nerves to degenerate and contributed to painful and progressive ulcerations of her legs and feet. She also was badly injured in a traffic accident in which her pelvis and a foot were crushed. Her polio, congenital spinal condition, and accident caused health problems throughout her life and resulted in numerous operations.

In *The Two Fridas* (Figure 8.3), Kahlo painted herself as two people: one Frida is dressed as a bride, and the other wears a Mexican costume. Both Fridas are connected through their hearts by a thin red artery that drips blood on the bridal gown. Kahlo's image conveys the experience of a woman trying to control a life tormented by continuous physical pain and shows that the serenity of the two faces is merely a façade that barely conceals her real suffering. In other paintings, Kahlo shows herself crying or suffering with pain, creating images of her body lacerated with nails, and, in one well-known work, she paints her spine as a broken pillar.

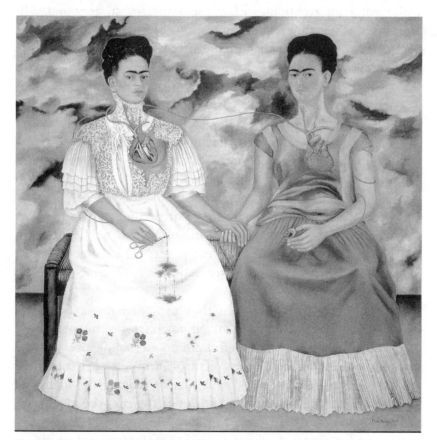

Figure 8.3 *The Two Fridas*, by Frida Kahlo
(Reprinted with permission of the National Institute for Belle Arts and Literature, Mexico, Permission no. 104/98. From Museo de Arte Moderno Collection.)

Artist Paul Klee is remembered for his playful and lively paintings and drawings. However, he suffered in the second half of his life from a condition known as scleroderma, a progressive disease that causes the shrinkage of skin and muscles, and as a result, he found it difficult to create detailed pictures. Many of his later works show his struggle both physically and emotionally with the course of his illness. Klee noted during this period, "Never have I drawn so much nor so intensely . . . I create in order not to cry."

Darcy Lynn is a contemporary artist who used art making to confront and cope with serious and life-threatening illness. Lynn, diagnosed with lymphoma in April 1991, found strength and hope through painting. She used her paintings to explore her experiences with medical interventions, such as chemotherapy, surgery, and radiation to treat her cancer; her impressions of hospitals and medical personnel; and her adjustment to life after lymphoma. She describes her experience as follows:

> Artists have always used their creative talents to help them deal with life's difficulties. I never found this to be more true than when I was stricken with lymphoma in April 1991. My circumstances were such that I was diagnosed only after life-saving surgery and chemotherapy.
>
> I spent three weeks in the hospital, was released for three weeks, and was readmitted with an unidentified lung infection. I was kept on IV antibiotics, and a Hickman catheter was inserted into a vein in my chest to facilitate the administration of the antibiotics and, of course, the chemotherapy.
>
> During my two stays in the hospital, I managed to draw and make sketches of myself, my doctors, and images I had either seen or invented. I am an eternal daydreamer and have always composed pictures in my head. I found that it relieved the stress while in the hospital. I finally applied my ideas to paint in mid-June after my second stay in the hospital. I was able to paint a few hours each day except for chemo days and when I was too fatigued or ill.
>
> Painting provided the one control I had of my situation. No one could tell me how or what to paint! Doctors controlled my body, but I controlled my soul. Painting offered

me a world of my making—an escape from the angst, yet, at the same time, a way for me to show myself what was happening and how strong I was. I was very fortunate to have the encouragement of my family, friends, and doctors in creating the work. They understood its importance.

I learned much from my illness, most importantly the need to be true to myself. I have continued to paint with as much passion and intensity as I felt during that time. For me, having had lymphoma freed a whole side of my personality that otherwise might never have emerged. I have always known the value of being an artist. Now I have confirmation and a larger canvas upon which to create.

In Lynn's painting *Rebirth* (Figure 8.4), the artist conveys her experience of overcoming a life-threatening illness. She says:

Rebirth is about all the new and positive changes that happened to me as a result of the cancer. I was completely bald, head and body, and felt reborn. A feeling of newness spread

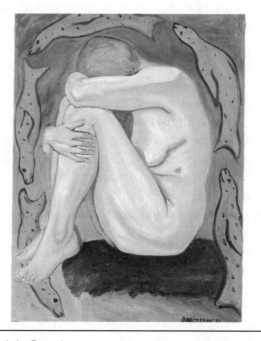

Figure 8.4 *Rebirth,* by Darcy Lynn   *(Reprinted with permission of the artist)*

through me, and felt like a child/woman starting over. I had an appreciation of my body and soul and felt blessed for seeing how wonderful life is. The seals swim around like angels flying. The painting is about the realization that life is a gift, and the image became such a positive one for me that seals became my motif for survival and hope.

Lynn's experience demonstrates the compelling power of art expression when one is confronting issues of life and death. Her paintings express feelings about illness that are difficult to communicate through words. Illness is a frightening, sometimes contradictory experience that is inevitably infused with feelings of crisis and pain. Although sickness is perceived as inherently negative in Western culture, images allow us to see disease and physical disability in a somewhat different light. Art helps us understand the emotional and spiritual aspects that come with confronting the loss of one's health.

Creativity and Health

Engaging in the process of creating art may actually produce positive physical changes in the body. With the continued interest in alternative and complementary forms of treatment, there is a renewed attention to how the body and mind connect and communicate with one another. Brain scans show increased blood flow to the brain during periods of creative thought, and any creative activity that is enjoyable gives rise to alpha wave patterns typical of restful alertness, the relaxed but aware state found in meditation. Serotonin, the chemical that alleviates feelings of depression, is also increased during creative activity. Therapeutic art programs in hospitals have been found to provide many benefits, including reduction of stress, increased capacity to communicate feelings about symptoms, and improvement of blood pressure, heart rate, and respiration.

Finally, creative experiences are known to enhance brain functioning and structure, perhaps even into old age. Gene Cohen, an authority on creativity and aging, observes that through creative self-expression, older individuals can actually increase the number of connections among brain cells, including those for memory and reaction. According to Cohen, creativity challenges people to increase their abilities and offers the possibility of a longer, more active life span. Engaging in activities such as painting or sculpting, along with having a positive outlook, boosts the immune system and may even eliminate depressive and sleep disorders believed to be a natural outcome of aging.

The Power of Opening Up in Health and Well-Being

Chapter 7 demonstrated how art can be useful in expressing feelings and recovering from emotional trauma. In most circumstances, art therapy is used to help people open up, to make visible their thoughts, feelings, and perceptions through drawing, painting, and other art forms. The goal of opening up is to help people understand the source of emotional distress or trauma and to alleviate and resolve conflicts.

Opening up through art expression can also contribute to health and wellness, and sharing powerful or disturbing feelings is known to contribute to overall physical well-being. We are all familiar with the stressful effects of holding on to anger, anxiety, or grief. Unexpressed, these feelings can have harmful effects on the body, such as heart disease, chronic pain, or immune dysfunction. Research on the impact of expressing traumatic experiences underscores its health-giving benefits, including increased immunity and the need for fewer visits to a doctor.

Because art serves as a way to open up about feelings, it provides health care professionals with information about their patients. From his experiences with cancer patients of all ages, Bernie Siegel observes that drawing is an easy and reliable way to reveal otherwise unexpressed feelings and beliefs. To help him understand his patients' perceptions of their cancer, he asks them to make a few very simple drawings depicting themselves, their treatment, their disease, and their white cells eliminating the disease, as well as an additional drawing of anything they choose. He uses drawing to help people open up and talk about feelings or experiences they might not otherwise share. For example, a drawing may be extremely helpful in revealing a patient's unexpressed conflicts about treatment. While a person may say that chemotherapy is helpful in eliminating his or her cancer, on an unconscious level the person may be feeling that the treatment is poison. These unrecognized beliefs, emotions, and perceptions about illness and medical interventions are important in developing an appropriate medical program for the patient.

People who are seriously ill often have two explanations for their condition, one spoken and one unspoken. The spoken one is a description of their condition based on knowledge of the physical aspects of medical diagnosis and treatment. The other, the unspoken one, is a more personal and often private perception of their illness. This personal explanation may or may not be conscious and may involve apprehension, confusion, misunderstanding, fear, and/or anxiety. It is often more likely to be revealed through art rather than communicated with words. For example, a nine-year-old child who was about to have surgery for a tumor cheerfully awaited the procedure and was even able to reassure her parents and siblings that everything would be all right. In a spontaneous drawing she did for me just before surgery, she depicted herself as a small figure standing next to a black figure (Figure 8.5). When I

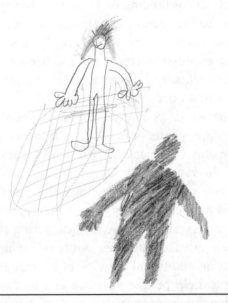

Figure 8.5 A nine-year-old girl's drawing before surgery
(Reprinted from Understanding Children's Drawings © 1998 Cathy A. Malchiodi, Guilford Publications)

asked her to tell me about the drawing, particularly the black figure, she said that this was a ghost and he told her in a dream that she was going to die. Although her surgery went extremely well and her prognosis for a full recovery was excellent, the girl's drawing conveyed unexpressed fears that she would die. Art opened a way for her to communicate the apprehension that she felt uncomfortable about expressing with words.

With another patient, art allowed the expression of anxieties that might otherwise have been left unsaid. Beth depicted the unpredictable and confusing nature of her cancer through an image of herself between life and death (Figure 8.6). She described herself as "standing alone between worlds":

> Death on the left. Life on the right. Bracing against both and not knowing which path, direction I'm going. The battle is not with Death because that is inevitable but maybe for Life. Both take a lot of energy—life and death. Both are bridges that are painful and confusing. But my feet are planted on flowing waters that lead me to where I am supposed to go. And outside of it all I see light and loving arms that will lead me home.

Beth's image communicated her struggle with a life-threatening illness and illuminated her feelings about moving between living and dying. Her image also reinforced and expressed her spiritual beliefs, something that sustained her through the difficult months of chemotherapy and radiation treatment.

Art Therapy in Medical Settings

Art therapy has been used in a variety of ways with people of all ages who are physically ill, experiencing pain or other chronic symptoms, or undergoing medical treatment such as surgery or drug interventions. It is used for many reasons, including psychotherapy to help patients cope with emotional distress, integrate experiences, and express feelings about illness or medical procedures. For example, an art therapist might provide children with activities in the preoperative room to encourage them to express feelings and to

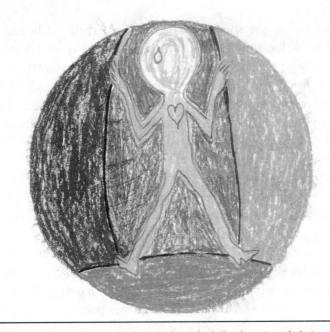

Figure 8.6 A drawing by Beth, a cancer survivor, depicting her struggle between life and death

explore their perceptions of their bodies and weight gain. A counselor might use art therapy to help a support group for cancer survivors communicate reactions to life-threatening illness and to share experiences with other patients. Or a therapist may use drawing along with relaxation exercises to help a person control or overcome headaches, reduce back pain, or imagine a stronger immune system.

Art therapy may also be used in rehabilitation programs where people are recovering from accidents, surgery, or acute and chronic conditions. An art therapist may develop a program in a long-term-care facility for elderly patients who are recovering from strokes or other illnesses or work with people who have orthopedic problems or head injuries due to an accident. The therapist may design art activities not only to enhance self-expression and creativity but also to help patients acquire skills or relearn dexterity. The following example describes one of many ways in which art therapy is used with medical populations.

A Medical Art Therapist at Work

Psychologist and art therapist Robin Gabriels uses art as a way to understand and evaluate children and adolescents with severe asthma. Her work at National Jewish Hospital in Denver convinced her that drawings are an important form of expression for this population, particularly because many of these young patients have a difficult time using words to express their feelings about their illness.

Gabriels asked patients to draw three pictures about their asthma. In the first picture, they were asked to draw what it feels like to have an asthma attack. Next, they were asked to draw a "helpful or good" environment, either real or imaginary, in which they would not have to worry about having asthma attacks. Finally, they were asked to depict a "harmful or bad" environment, either real or imaginary, in which they would be plagued by asthma attacks. After completing each drawing, the children had the opportunity to discuss their pictures; they often revealed many of their fears, concerns, and perceptions of their illness.

Fifteen-year-old Jamie was referred for art therapy because of emotional problems that exacerbated her asthma. In her first picture, she drew herself trapped under water and unable to breathe (Figure 8.7). According to Gabriels, this image revealed much more of Jamie's anxiety, pain, and fear about her condition than she was able to verbalize. In her "helpful or good" environment drawing, Jamie depicted herself in a balloon, a place where she was protected from environmental things that could trigger her asthma (Figure 8.8). Jamie included another person, who holds the balloon; Gabriels notes that this perhaps reflects her wish to let someone else care for her.

In her last picture, Jamie represented a "bad" environment as a hill on which she was alone (Figure 8.9). The picture depicted things that triggered her asthma: grasses, humidity, and emotions. Jamie stated that she was holding a snake, which caused her to feel anxious—anxiety being another trigger for her asthma attacks.

These drawings were useful in developing a plan of treatment for Jamie and explaining to Jamie's father her perceptions and fears about her asthma. Gabriels notes that this process of drawing helps

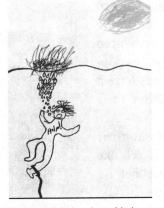

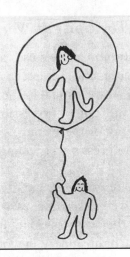

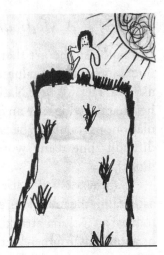

Figure 8.7 A drawing of being trapped under water and unable to breathe, by Jamie, a girl with asthma
(Reprinted with permission from Dr. Robin Gabriels)

Figure 8.8 A drawing of a "helpful/good" environment, by Jamie
(Reprinted with permission from Dr. Robin Gabriels)

Figure 8.9 A drawing of a "bad" environment, by Jamie
(Reprinted with permission from Dr. Robin Gabriels)

children cope with their illness by identifying and expressing their feelings about it. It also helps the therapist understand the child's experience.

Art in Hospitals

Because of the recognition of the therapeutic powers of art expression, there is an increasing use of arts in all forms in hospital settings. Visual artists, along with musicians, poets, storytellers, and dancers, are being used in more and more hospitals all the time. They assist patients in making art either at the bedside or in groups. These art programs may not provide psychotherapy, but they clearly have therapeutic value. Many are designed to improve patient morale and to enhance the healing process. Others are intended to provide arts medicine, a philosophy described in Chapter 2.

Tracy Council, an art therapist at Georgetown University in Washington, D.C., provides art activities and other creative experiences for young cancer patients. The purpose of the program is to encourage patients to use art activities to express feelings about their illnesses and medical interventions as well as to provide an experience of normalcy through creative expression. Council inspires her patients to enhance their hospital rooms with their own self-created mobiles, tabletop fountains, and wall art in order to help in relaxation and to distract them from painful procedures. Annual pediatric art exhibits featuring children's drawings, paintings, and sculptures, as well as group art projects, increase patients' self-esteem and affirm that their creative potential is acknowledged and appreciated.

The purpose of art programs in hospitals varies widely. In some programs, interaction with patients and their families is emphasized, while in others, the impact of the aesthetic qualities of art is the primary consideration. For example, art by local artists may be used to enhance the hospital's environment by being exhibited in waiting rooms or patient areas to create a more visually pleasing interior. In some facilities, artists have designed "healing environments"—interiors designed to calm and relax patients and their families.

Although art programs, exhibitions, and specially designed interiors are not always defined as art therapy, many aspects of this use of art in hospitals are therapeutic. Making art within the confines of a hospital room can improve quality of life and provide meaningful activity during long hours of boredom or recovery. Exposure to paintings, sculptures, or other art forms certainly can be normalizing within an environment usually devoid of aesthetic aspects. Although healing environments created to calm and relax patients and their families may or may not have the effect the artist intended, they unquestionably improve the quality of care within medical settings.

Guided Imagery and Drawing

Guided imagery, or guided visualization, a series of directives to use one's mind to imagine various scenes or events in a relaxed state, has become increasingly popular used in conjunction with the treatment of cancer and other diseases. You may be familiar with the variety of available audiotapes that use guided imagery to help people relieve stress, control pain, stop smoking, or lose weight. The term *visualization*, which is sometimes used interchangeably with the term *guided imagery*, simply refers to the formation of mental pictures or the conscious creation of images. There are two types of visualizations: receptive, in which participants develop their own images, and programmed, in which individuals respond to guided imagery created for a specific purpose, such as pain reduction, symptom relief, or healing. Over the past several decades, the use of imagery has become an important topic in complementary and traditional medicine, and a number of researchers are investigating the possible links between mental imagery and physical health.

Guided visualizations have been specifically designed to treat illness or medical conditions, to induce relaxation and reduce stress, to alleviate depression, and to enhance sports performance. The best-known guided visualizations designed to treat illness were developed by Carl Simonton and Stephanie Matthews, who have used imagery exercises with people with cancer since the 1970s. Simonton, a radiologist, believes that patients can benefit through mental imagery and relaxation and that regular use of guided imagery can stimulate the immune system and help patients feel that they are active participants in their medical treatment. Psychologist Jeanne Achterburg has investigated the use of imagery with people with a wide variety of illnesses and conditions and has developed a series of guided visualizations for specific symptoms and diseases. The widespread use of visualization with cancer patients and people with HIV or AIDS or other serious illnesses has established the value and power of imagery to alter body reactions, sensations, and responses. Studies point to the possibility that proper use of visualization may even extend the life span of the seriously ill and, at the very least, decrease perceptions of pain or other symptoms.

Guided visualization is thought to benefit those people with chronic or life-threatening illnesses in several ways. First, imagery affects attitude. It can reduce depression, anxiety, and negative thinking, which in turn can enhance healing. Imagery combined with relaxation techniques can lower blood pressure and can slow heart rate. Imagery can also alleviate the side effects of drugs, including those used in chemotherapy.

Because art therapy involves the use of imagery, it is sometimes confused with guided imagery. Art therapists often use guided imagery, and professionals who use guided imagery with their patients sometimes use drawing, asking people to create a picture after leading them through a specific experience with guided imagery. For example, Carl Simonton, Jeanne Achterburg, and Bernie Siegel have all asked people to visualize and draw their medical treatment (chemotherapy, radiation, or other interventions) successfully eliminating their cancer. Many therapists use guided imagery along with art expression to help people relax, reduce stress, alleviate depression and anxiety, and reduce symptoms of disease or pain.

I use several simple guided-imagery exercises with people who want to enhance their health or ameliorate a medical condition or symptom. Each visualization should be preceded by a relaxation exercise, such as the one described at the end of Chapter 4. You may also want to draw your experience after trying each of these exercises, using colors, images, and sensations to record your feelings and any changes you sense in your body.

Use Color to Soothe Your Symptoms

Think about your favorite colors or color scheme, and imagine those colors in the form of a beam of light. In your imagination, direct the beam of light to the areas where you need relief. If you have trouble visualizing your favorite colors, you might want to try to imagine a white or golden light pouring through your body. You can also try selecting a warm color (such as red) or a cool color (such as blue) to warm or cool the area of your body.

After completing this exercise, try making a drawing of the colors you used in your visualization or sketch any sensations of color that you imagined or felt. You may want to use a copy of the body image template described a little later in this chapter to record your experiences of color.

Imagine an Outside Source of Healing

Try mentally picturing the part of the body that needs attention (for example, your back, if you have back pain). Think of what that area of your body needs, such as warmth, coolness, or relief of tension. Now try to imagine what might provide that relief, such as sunlight, gentle water, or healing hands. For example, a person suffering from shoulder pain might try visualizing warm sunlight bathing and penetrating that part of the body. In your mind's eye, see the source of relief coming to your injured or ill body part. Imagine it soothing and alleviating your symptoms.

Use a Positive Image of Health or Recovery

Try imagining yourself in optimal condition, seeing yourself engaged in a favorite activity or sport and participating without pain, discomfort, or worry. Visualize yourself as symptom free as possible, seeing yourself active, energetic, and joyful. What things give you pleasure and vitality in life? Try to see yourself in situations that give you happiness, energy, or inspiration. Follow up your visualization by selecting collage images from magazines that capture an image of health (see the Symbol of Health activity a little later in this chapter). Glue these images on a piece of paper or cardboard, and hang your collage somewhere where you can see it each day and reflect on what gives you positive and healthy feelings.

These are just a few of the ways you can use mental imagery to enhance health and well-being. Guided imagery and visualization require practice on a regular basis and are more effective when repeated at least twice a day for ten to twenty minutes. They also work best just before falling asleep, possibly because most people are in a very relaxed state at that time of the day. Creating art images of your guided imagery or visualization experiences can reinforce the mental images you develop to enhance well-being and may deepen your understanding of how imagery can specifically help in healing or relieving symptoms.

Using Art Making for Health and Well-Being

In addition to visualization, the following activities may be helpful in addressing and working on issues of health and well-being through art making.

Body Drawing

Materials: body image template and oil pastels, colored pencils, or felt markers

1. Make several copies of the body image template (Figure 8.10) in this chapter. If you want to work within a larger format, have the template enlarged by a copy store or simply make your own body drawing on a large piece of white paper. Use a pencil or black felt-tip marker to make a simple outline similar to the one provided.
2. Spend a couple of minutes with your eyes closed, noticing how your body feels. Start from your feet and work your way up your body, making a mental note of any sensations, tension, pain, or other feelings in different areas of your body.
3. Use colored drawing materials to fill in your body image with colors, lines, and shapes (Figure 8.11). Try to do this spontaneously and intuitively, and don't worry about being

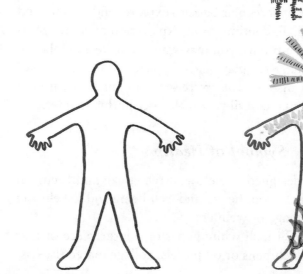

Figure 8.10 Body image template

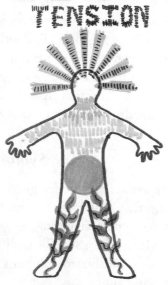

Figure 8.11 An example of the body image exercise, showing tension

realistic. Your goal is to represent feelings about your body rather than actual characteristics. You may also draw around the outside of the body image, using colors, lines, and shapes to complete any areas you feel the need to.

After you finish your drawing, write a few phrases or words describing your image. Think about how you used colors, lines, or shapes throughout the body outline. If you depicted a specific symptom, sensation, tension, or pain, try answering the following questions about your drawing:

- Where is the symptom (pain, swelling, itchiness, wound, inflammation, and so on) the greatest? For example, if you have pain in a specific part of your body, where is it the most painful?
- Does the pain or other symptom have a specific shape and color?
- Are there any other sensations present in your body, and how did you depict them through colors, lines, or shapes?

Many patients who have an ongoing physical illness or condition use this exercise on a regular basis to explore, understand, and cope with symptoms. To continue your exploration of body sensations, feelings, and symptoms, you may want to make a number of copies of the body image template and complete one or two images each week. You may also use this exercise in conjunction with the somatic drawing journal described a little later in this chapter.

Symbol of Health

This art activity is designed to help you recognize and focus on things that contribute to your health and well-being and to help you develop a personal image of wellness.

Materials: 18 × 24 inch white paper or a large piece of mat board or cardboard, felt pens or oil pastels, collage materials, scissors, and glue

1. Take a few minutes to think about what makes you feel healthy or contributes to your health or well-being. Consider that health and well-being come from many sources: physical, emotional, social, and spiritual aspects of life. Try answering the following questions:
   - Are there activities that contribute to your feeling physically healthy?
   - What emotional relationships give you pleasure or support you?
   - What kinds of social support (church, school, family, friends, and so on) are present in your life?
   - Do you have beliefs that sustain your spiritual side?
   - Are there any changes or additions to these aspects of your life that you would like to make?

   Consider how all these elements support your overall health, and write down some of the images or ideas that come to mind.

2. Using any or all of the materials, create a picture that contains images you think contribute to your health. You can also add elements that may not be currently present in your life but that you think would add to your overall health and well-being. You can create this image on a sheet of white paper or cut out a large circle on paper, mat board, or cardboard, using it to draw on or to attach collage materials.

   When you have completed your symbol, place or hang it in an area of your art-making space or home where you can see it on a regular basis. Many people I see in my art therapy practice place the symbols of health they have created in a prominent place in their homes or offices in order to reinforce ideas and experiences that they find healing. Others have created their symbols on a form similar to a shield, which they take to chemotherapy, radiation, or hospital stays. Try using your symbol to reinforce the images in your life that contribute to your health, and add to it as new images and ideas emerge.

Creating a Healthy Place

Most children and adults who have a serious or chronic physical condition not only need to identify healthy aspects of their lives but also need to explore self-care as a part of their health maintenance. While children really like this art activity, I find that adults enjoy it, too, because it involves an element of play.

For this exercise, you will need a plastic animal or another small figure, preferably one of an animal that you like. If you do not have one on hand, go to a toy store and purchase a bag of plastic farm or jungle animals.

Materials: a plastic animal or figure of your choice, 18 × 24 inch white paper, oil pastels, paint, collage materials, scissors, glue, and a cardboard box (optional)

1. Take a few minutes to meditate on the animal figure you have selected. Notice its characteristics and imagine what it would look like if it were life-size. Where would this animal live (jungle, rural area, forest, and so on)? What would it need to survive? To feel safe and comfortable? What would it need to feel well cared for and nurtured? Take a few more minutes and, with eyes closed, imagine an environment for this animal that would meet these needs.
2. With any of the materials, create this safe, comfortable, and nurturing environment for the animal. Use the animal figure as part of the actual art piece. You may want to use a sheet of white paper for the base or a cardboard box to contain your environment. Use drawing materials, paints, and/or collage materials to make the environment.

This exercise may take several sessions. People often find that there are elements they wish to add to their animal's environment. When you complete the exercise, write down your answers to the following questions:

- What items, surroundings, circumstances, or qualities are important to make your animal feel safe, comfortable, and nurtured?

- How did you decide what elements to include?
- Are there any elements you wanted to include but didn't?
- What helps you feel safe, comfortable, and nurtured?

Keeping a Somatic Drawing Journal

A somatic drawing journal is for creating images specifically about how your body feels. Select a journal or sketchbook for the type of materials (drawing, painting, or collage) you will be using to make images. You may also want to work with the body-image exercise over several weeks or months, particularly if you have a symptom or condition you want to monitor through images. By making a series of photocopies of the template and having them bound together into a book, you can make a body image journal in which to regularly record colors and shapes that relate to sensations in your body.

Relaxation or meditation can be an important part of your work with image making. Deep relaxation and meditation are known to lower blood pressure, pulse rate, and the level of stress hormones in the blood. Overall, reaching a relaxed state on a regular basis is thought to be important in health maintenance and to help people live longer and better lives. Although you do not have to start art making with relaxation, I tell people who have a medical condition that it can't hurt to include it as part of their creative process of visual journaling.

Drawing physical symptoms in your somatic journal over time can be helpful for several reasons. First, you will record your physical sensations and be able to observe how they change. This can be particularly important if you are experiencing chronic pain, nausea, dizziness, or other symptoms that change during the course of weeks or months or occur only at certain times. When I was chronically ill several years ago, I found that drawing my pain and other symptoms over several weeks helped me understand what might be triggering symptoms. It also was helpful information to share with my doctor and helped him to narrow down causes for my symptoms.

Jane Berstein, an artist and art therapist, used her own form of a somatic visual journal to record, understand, and cope with endometriosis, an extremely painful pelvic condition that is difficult to diagnose and treat. Over the course of twelve years, Berstein created approximately 450 drawings, discovering that making images was helpful even when doctors missed diagnosing her illness. She also shared the drawings with some of the doctors she saw while being treated. As a result of documenting her experience with endometriosis through drawing, Berstein found a personal visual language for her pain.

In addition to making images relating to feelings and/or symptoms, you might want to try recording dreams in the form of drawings in your somatic journal. I often ask people who come to my practice about their dreams, particularly if they have a physical illness. Through noticing and recording dream images and feelings about dreams, people with physical illness may learn more about their condition and what is happening within their bodies. For example, Peter, a thirty-eight-year-old man with HIV, realized through keeping a journal of the images in his dreams that his dreams of spinning and falling predicted that he was about to get an infection. He would generally see himself in these dreams caught in a tornado, spinning in circles and falling into the vortex. Peter used the visual journal I asked him to work on between art therapy sessions to record his dream images and found them to be helpful in monitoring his health.

Drawing physical symptoms can provide a sense of control rather than feeling victimized by an illness or condition. One important predictive aspect of health and recovery is the ability to feel that one has an internal sense of control. Using a journal to explore and express experiences with illness, medical treatment, or symptoms will not completely restore stamina, autonomy, or health, but a journal that is used on a regular basis can help support an internal sense of strength, capability, and mastery.

Finally, consider any or all of the following questions after completing each drawing in your journal:

- If you could talk with your image, what would it say to you?
- Is there something that your image wants to do?
- If you have a specific symptom, such as pain, fever, or another discomfort, how does it feel? What colors, lines, shapes, or themes have you used to describe it?

- What don't you like about your symptom or illness? What do you like about it?
- What colors, lines, shapes, or content would make your symptoms or illness feel better? Try making an additional drawing that depicts these elements.

Art created at times of crisis can be quite powerful, revelatory, and even mysterious. It is important for you to be connected to others for emotional assistance, whether it comes from a therapist, medical personnel, or a support group. The latter, support groups, can also be a way to explore the healing powers of art making and the creative process and are the subject of the next chapter.

9

Art Therapy Groups: Drawing Together

ART MAKING IS traditionally a solitary activity. When you think of art making, you generally think of an individual working alone in a studio, a place that is separate from the rest of the world. Because art making is a self-absorbing and personal activity, it is natural to think that one would be alone to make art.

Art has probably been made by groups of people since the dawn of human history. Healing rituals frequently involve support and the presence of a group or community of individuals and often involve imagery as part of the experience. For example, the Navajo people create elaborate sandpaintings for specific healing purposes, and, as part of the process, family and friends gather to witness and participate in the event. Visual objects and images are often used by groups to honor, commemorate, or make closure with a death or memorable experience. You may remember the end of the movie *Schindler's List*, when survivors and their descendants filed past the grave, each leaving a stone on the tomb. The AIDS Memorial Quilt is another powerful example of how people have used art to express feelings of grief and loss as well as to create a visual legacy of someone they have loved.

The practice of art therapy often takes place in groups. Many hospitals have art therapy programs or arts medicine programs that provide art-making opportunities for groups of people who have mental or physical illnesses. Clinics, community agencies, and shelters also offer art therapy groups for a variety of individuals, including survivors of trauma, people with alcoholism or drug dependencies, and individuals with serious or life-threatening illnesses, such as cancer or AIDS. Many of these programs are conducted by art therapists, psychologists, social workers, or counselors, while others are led by artists in residence who develop and conduct art studios for patients.

In psychiatric hospital settings, most art therapy takes place in groups. Often people work individually on their own art within the group, creating either spontaneous or nondirected art expressions, while others may be directed by a therapist to create an art piece around a theme or an idea.

Curative Potential of Art Therapy Groups

While art making on your own can be fulfilling, therapeutic, and healing, art making within a group offers some special qualities. Irving Yalom, a psychiatrist respected for his work with groups, believes that there are curative factors found in groups. Some of these include the following:

- **Instilling hope.** Art therapy with groups involves being part of a supportive community of people. This experience of group support and sharing naturally instills hope, particularly when group members relate positive experiences of overcoming or solving problems and talk about their own recovery from trauma, loss, illness, family conflicts, or addictions.
- **Interaction.** Groups provide the opportunity for social interaction. More important, they provide social support, which has been connected to health and well-being. Art making within a group connects group members with each other through group projects and/or through the sharing of art made during the session.
- **Universality.** Groups show participants that others have similar problems, worries, and fears and that people's experiences are more similar than different. While

experiences may be universal, images people create also may carry universal meaning, but in a very personal or unique way. Sharing common symbols and/or experiences is an important function of an art therapy group and reduces isolation through communication and exchange of mutual concerns.

- **Catharsis.** As with individual art therapy, group work can be particularly helpful in catharsis and expression of painful feelings or experiences. Catharsis within a supportive group is reported to be helpful in overcoming distressful or traumatic events and in sharing anxieties, fears, depression, and other emotions that result from grief and loss.

- **Altruism.** Group therapy emphasizes helping one another through difficult times. This sense of altruism can be a healing factor for the person who gives help as well as for the one who receives it. Art therapy groups encourage support between group members by offering creative activities through which people can interact in positive and helpful ways.

These curative characteristics apply to most art therapy groups, and a therapist may capitalize on any or all of these healing potentials through art experientials.

While many types of art therapy groups exist, there are basically two kinds: art psychotherapy groups and art studio or open studio groups. Many groups are a mixture of both philosophies, depending on the needs of group members, the goals of the experience, and the context or setting for the group.

Art Psychotherapy Groups

An art psychotherapy group is usually designed to help people express feelings, problems, or conflicts; achieve insight; or resolve painful emotions or experiences. Art psychotherapy groups came about in the 1960s, at approximately the same time that encounter and other types of groups were popular. They may emphasize individual art-making experiences within the group or focus more on group dynamics, interaction, and communication between group members through art activities.

In an art psychotherapy group, the therapist often takes an active role in determining themes and directives, designing group art activities with particular goals in mind. These are based on what the therapist has observed about the participants or what the participants determine is important to explore. For example, group members may be asked to identify problems or themes that they would like to explore through art. In my work as an art therapist with a breast cancer support group, participants wanted to explore and communicate issues about medical treatments for cancer and its effects on their bodies. With this in mind, we created an eight-week art therapy support group, which met once a week to participate in an art activity developed by the women and myself. Each week, we selected a different theme to use as a focus for art making and discussion. The themes included staying well (making a symbol of health), hospital life (creating group murals depicting staying at the hospital), and body image after cancer (designing life-size body images exploring postmastectomy thoughts and feelings). Using themes in art therapy groups provides a focus for art making and a structure for participation and helps the group to become cohesive more quickly.

Art psychotherapy groups are often formed around a specific population. For example, you might encounter an art psychotherapy group for parents whose children are seriously ill, recovering alcoholics, women who have been battered by their spouses, children who have been abused, or teenagers with behavioral problems. Some art psychotherapy groups may also serve as support groups, such as for individuals with HIV or AIDS, people who are grieving the loss of a family member, children of alcoholics, or breast cancer survivors.

Some art psychotherapy groups emphasize interaction among group members through shared art making. This type of group focuses on the actions and reactions of participants to each other while engaged in art making and encourages members to respond to the content of each other's participation and artwork. Art therapists who use this approach may help group members to identify distorted perceptions or assumptions, interpersonal beliefs and actions, and patterns of interaction with other individuals. Family art therapy, described a little later in the chapter, uses many of the same principles as interactive art psychotherapy.

Art psychotherapy groups may be time limited; that is, they may meet regularly for a certain number of sessions, a daylong intensive, or, in some cases, only one or two sessions. In a hospital, the group may meet regularly, but the participants may change because people in that setting come and go frequently. Groups may also meet for different lengths of time, anywhere from an hour to three hours depending on the context, the objectives of the group, and the participants.

Most art psychotherapy groups follow a similar format, including an opening discussion, an experiential process, and a postexperiential discussion. In the first part of the session, the therapist may introduce the theme or activity of the group. In some groups, the participants use this time to develop a directive or theme with help from the therapist for experiential work. In nondirective groups, the participants may be working on ongoing projects, such as painting, drawings, mixed media, or constructions.

During the middle part of an art psychotherapy group, participants make images in response to a theme or a directive (for example, "Draw yourself as an animal" or "Create a symbol of health"). In some circumstances, the therapist designs activities in which a group of people can experience working together on the same art piece, rather than each making individual images. For example, a group of adolescents might be provided with a large circle drawn on paper and asked to imagine what they could include within the circle if it were a world. The group would then work together, with the therapist's guidance, to select images or draw pictures within the circle that represent ideas related to the theme.

Following the art activity, there is usually a group discussion. Each participant may talk for a few minutes about the image he or she made during the session or share his or her impressions of the group experience. If there was a particular theme for the group, participants may discuss their work as it relates to that theme.

For the therapist and participants, a collaborative work of art such as a large drawing or mural may help in understanding and exploring group dynamics. Group situations naturally create the opportunity for communication, interaction, negotiation, and other types of exchange. The therapist may choose to illuminate some of the group dynamics that took place during the art activity, such as who took the leadership role, who directed the activity, and how well the group worked together. Participants may express what feelings came up for them in making decisions about creating art together, or they may discuss the content of the finished work.

An Art Psychotherapy Group for Survivors of Child Sexual Abuse

Survivors of childhood sexual abuse often struggle with the effects of trauma for many years, even into adulthood. They may experience emotional difficulties, including depression and posttraumatic stress disorder (PTSD), and reactions, such as anxiety, fear, nightmares, or helplessness. Many sexual-abuse survivors do not remember their abuse, having repressed memories of their experiences. Carla, whom I described in an earlier chapter, was sexually abused as a child but did not remember the details of her abuse until, as a young adult, she began to have recurrent and intrusive memories and dreams about her experiences. As a result, she began drawing images of her memories and recollections about her childhood abuse.

Sexual-abuse survivors in this particular group were women between the ages of thirty-two and fifty-four and were in treatment for anxiety, depression, and other emotional difficulties that resulted from unresolved issues of early abuse when they were children. The group took place over an eight-week period and met at a community mental health center for ninety-minute sessions. Women who were sexually abused as children and who came to the center for counseling were asked if they also would like to participate in group art therapy (in addition to their regular counseling) to explore their feelings and experiences with sexual abuse. None of the group members had ever participated in art therapy before, but they wanted to be part of a support group in which they could express and discuss issues relevant to childhood abuse with other women who'd had similar experiences.

While many art therapy groups do not have a weekly structure, because of the needs of the participants and the context of the group it was decided that weekly themes for directives would be developed. These themes were designed with the mental health agency's overall goals for the women in mind. The themes included expressing feelings through color and shape, making drawings of family of origin (the family into which a person is born and grows up in), creating a safe place, and exploring feelings about the perpetrator. Because the group was time limited and the women in the group had little or no experience with art, simple materials, such as felt markers, collage materials, and oil pastels, were offered. (See Figure 9.1.)

While it is impossible to fully describe the week-by-week process of the art psychotherapy group for these survivors of childhood

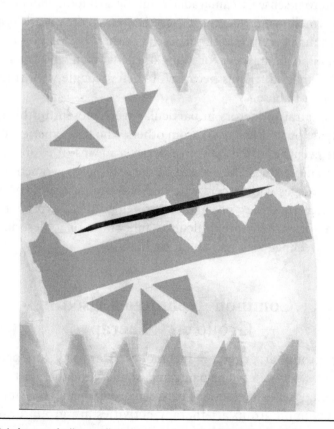

Figure 9.1 *Anger*, a feelings collage by a survivor of childhood sexual abuse

abuse, some of the women's observations of the art therapy process underscore the importance and value of group art therapy. In the beginning, sharing was difficult, but art making made the process easier for most of the group members. Several women remarked that art was especially helpful because they were told as children not to talk about their abuse; art, a natural form of communication during childhood, served as a safe way to communicate events that were kept secret for many years. Some women felt that art activities let them reclaim positive parts of their childhood, such as the ability to play, experiment, and create in a supportive environment. These parts were lost or forgotten and replaced by memories and unresolved issues of betrayal and mistrust during their early years.

The play and creativity involved in group art making contributed to a sense of camaraderie among group members. Activities in which group members were encouraged to work together brought many members closer to each other. Decreasing isolation was an important aspect for many of the women who felt separate from family and friends because of their struggle with traumatic memories of abuse.

Two curative factors in particular were present in this group: the impact of social support from others who had experienced similar life events and the power of art as a means of expression for trauma and feelings. At the end of the group, the women felt that sharing images with others who had had similar experiences reinforced that they were not alone. Art helped them express feelings and memories that were difficult to talk about or to describe, particularly feelings they had about their abusers.

Common Techniques Used in Group Art Therapy

Many group art therapy techniques are used to encourage exchanges between participants and to allow the therapist to stimulate and observe interactions between group members. Among the more common group art therapy activities are group drawings, paintings, or collages and dyad drawings.

Group Drawings, Paintings, or Collages

The therapist might ask the group to create an image focusing on a specific theme or allow the group to choose its own theme for art making. For example, a group may be asked to create a joint mural in which participants depict themselves as their favorite animals or to create a group collage that portrays a "perfect world" (Figure 9.2). The art process serves as a catalyst for group interaction and is followed by a group discussion of the image and participants' observations of the group dynamics.

Dyad Drawings

The word *dyad* simply means "two"; a dyad drawing is one in which two people draw together within the same space. In working with children, I sometimes work with a child on the same paper, or I may ask a mother and her child to work together so that I can observe

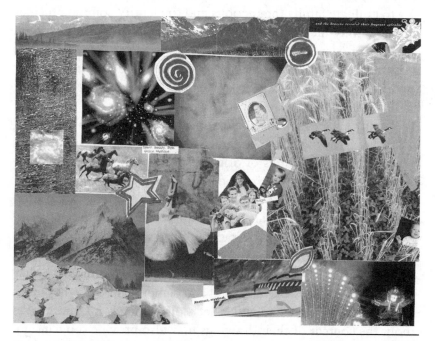

Figure 9.2 *Perfect World*, a group collage

their interactions. Other times I may ask two people to draw on the same sheet of paper but to do so without talking. This encourages a nonverbal "conversation" on paper. After a dyad drawing is completed, the therapist may ask the participants to talk about what they were thinking and feeling during the activity. In addition to drawing, a dyad might paint, sculpt, make a collage, or build something together.

Family Art Therapy

You may be surprised to learn that family art therapy is a popular way of working with parents, couples, and children within the context of a group. Family art therapy developed from art therapy and from the field of family therapy. Because families are essentially groups, family art therapy has similarities to other art psychotherapy groups. Family art therapy began in the 1960s and 1970s when art therapist Hanna Yaxa Kwiatkowska used a series of art activities to evaluate family interactions and to identify common themes among family members. Her work with families at the National Institute of Mental Health led to the growth and development of family art therapy techniques at about the same time that family therapy was becoming a popular method of treatment throughout the United States.

Family art therapy may be used to help families explore any or all of the following: family interactions and communication styles between members, family of origin issues, past family history, current family problems, or individual family members. Art therapy may provide the family with a new experience of communication and expression and provide the therapist with the opportunity to view how family members interact with one another and solve problems. When confronted with a new situation (in this case, making drawings together), the family may respond in ways in which they react to new experiences in general and demonstrate how they interact to solve problems or make decisions. Images and narratives about the content of their drawings may also provide some insight into how each family member feels and how the family as a whole interacts with each other.

Family art therapy may be used in a variety of situations. In general, families come to therapy for help with a particular family member, often referred to as the identified patient. While the identified patient may be perceived to be in distress or creating problems for the family as a whole, it is usually true that the entire family is distressed. For example, family art therapy may be used with families coping with a handicapped member, a terminally ill child, an alcoholic parent, or a troubled adolescent. In each case, art therapy may be used to explore how family members feel about the identified patient, how each views the problem, and how each envisions a solution.

A benefit of using art therapy with families is its ability to provide an appropriate means of expression and communication for all family members. Children, for instance, may be intimidated or uninterested in traditional verbal therapy or counseling. Art expression may offer them a developmentally appropriate means of participating in therapy because art is a natural means of expression for children. In the following example of a family confronting and recovering from domestic violence, a brother and sister were effectively able to communicate their experiences of domestic violence through art and to participate as a family in meaningful activities designed to help them overcome trauma and loss.

A Family Art Therapist at Work

Nora, a young mother of a nine-year-old daughter and a five-year-old son, sought outpatient treatment at a local mental health center just after terminating her marriage of ten years. She had experienced abuse from her husband, and recently she had to be rescued by police during a violent altercation with her husband when she refused to get an abortion. He was hitting and choking her and kicking their children to keep them away. Their son attempted to defend his mother with his toy sword, and the daughter dialed 911. Nora requested help for herself and her children from the mental health center just after this violent incident.

Shirley Riley, an art therapist and marriage and family therapist, used art expression to help the family process their trauma and the grief involved in going through a divorce. The father refused to be part of the treatment, and his contact with the children was limited to brief visits. The therapy took place over several months and included addressing the family's loss through divorce, the violence experienced, and the reinvention of the family's roles after the ending of the marriage. The goals of family art therapy included increasing communication between Nora and her children and helping them adjust to the loss of a husband and father.

After several months of work, the therapist asked the family to choose and then create their favorite fairy tale. Nora and her children decided on "Little Red Riding Hood." Using clay and construction paper, they created a scene of Red Riding Hood in the forest. Their re-creation included Red Riding Hood in the center, Grandmother in the doorway of her home, the wolf in a doghouse, and the woodsman bravely defending Grandmother. Nora observed that she identified with Red Riding Hood, who, she said, "foolishly goes into the woods knowing that it is dangerous." The daughter created the figures of Grandmother and the wolf, and the son created the woodsman, who saved Grandmother and killed the wolf, just as the boy had bravely rushed into the fray with his toy sword to save his own mother from danger.

The task allowed the family to metaphorically reenact the roles that each played in the original violent incident. It also gave the family the opportunity to adjust the fairy tale they chose to suit their own needs and provided a safe way to explore a new ending to their violent tale. The therapist was able to suggest modifications through the story of Red Riding Hood, employing the fairy tale as a nonthreatening, indirect way to explore the trauma in their lives. Using simple materials, both Nora and her children were able to manipulate and rearrange the characters in the story and to relate their personal stories and feelings through art. It also allowed them the chance to confront the abuser (the father) in a safe manner through the character of the wolf. In this case, it may have been undesirable to include the father in the session because it would evoke fear in the family and violate restrictions placed on him by the court. However, through art he could safely become part of the therapy.

In a subsequent session, Riley asked Nora and her children to create an image of what they would like from a "good man." The intent was to help the family explore their feelings about men in general. To facilitate this process, the therapist drew a large outline of a person on a six-foot piece of paper and asked Nora to be in charge of placing various collage images, chosen by herself and the children, on the figure. Nora and her children were also encouraged to write statements on the figure, with the art therapist helping as the scribe for the youngest child. Through this exercise, a fantasy of a new mate and father emerged on paper.

In this case, the family filled the outline with healthy, positive images, including pictures of families having fun and engaging in relaxing activities. In addition to identifying characteristics that would constitute an ideal mate and father, the exercise allowed the therapist to observe how the mother and children worked together to make decisions and share ideas. Nora was helpful and generous with her children's choices of pictures, while maintaining her own role as the adult in charge and attending to her own needs. They were also able to discuss what behaviors and traits they chose to leave out because they had led to unhappiness in the family during the previous marriage. This aspect was particularly important to the therapist's understanding of the family, as it indicated that they had created a man significantly different from the violent man they had left.

In a final session, the therapist asked each person to make a drawing of what things would be like in one year, in ten years, and beyond. Nora and her children had addressed and confronted the issues involved in the trauma and losses they had experienced and were now ready to move on, plan their future, and establish a new identity as a family. In her image, Nora established the goals for her future, including looking forward to a new home life with her children and not dwelling on the past. The experience of creating an image of the future at this point in treatment helped the family to perceive themselves through a different lens, one that reinforced a positive sense of self and future. (See Figures 9.3 and 9.4.)

Clearly, in cases such as this, family art therapy is a long-term process, and one collage or drawing does not instantaneously solve complex issues. For Nora and her children, the use of art served several important purposes that would be difficult to achieve through strictly verbal means. Through the use of tasks that required group participation, the therapist was easily able to see how the family interacted by observing how they communicated, shared ideas, planned, and executed art activities. Lastly, some of the stress of talking about their traumatic experiences was alleviated through the use of less direct expression in metaphor and visual images.

Family Art Therapy Techniques

In most cases, a family art therapist designs an art task for the family based on their needs and the goals for therapy. In the case just described, Riley developed art tasks to help Nora and her children explore issues of domestic violence, trauma, loss, and reinventing their family after divorce. There are some common family art ther-

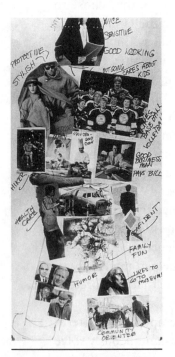

Figure 9.3 *An Ideal Mate/Father*, a group collage by Nora and her children

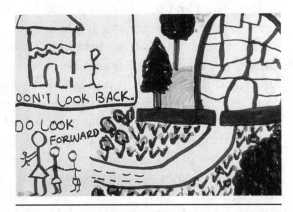

Figure 9.4 Nora's goals for the future

apy techniques that a therapist may use in work with families to evaluate communication between family members, to help with problem solving, or to encourage creative thinking.

Nonverbal Team Art Task

Art therapist Helen Landgarten describes a technique she calls a nonverbal team art task, an activity in which family members are asked to choose a partner within the family and create a joint drawing on the same piece of paper. For example, in a family of four (two parents and two sons), a mother and the oldest son may be one team, and the father and the youngest son may be the other team. Each team is told to create a picture without talking or signaling one another during the drawing. After they have completed the images, participants may talk to each other to come up with titles for their drawings.

Family Drawing or Collage

For this task, the family is given a large piece of paper on which to do a drawing or collage together. The task may be nonverbal or verbal (that is, family members may or may not be permitted to talk with each other during the process), and the therapist may assign a theme, such as "Draw yourselves living together on an island," or the subject matter of the artwork may be left up to the family. The therapist may guide the family in group work on their drawing or collage and usually interviews the family about their impressions of their experience after they have completed the image. Depending on the context and purpose of the art activity, the therapist may emphasize understanding the content and meaning of the image or the process and dynamics between family members.

Genograms

Family therapy often addresses ways in which individual family members interact and connect with each other. Family therapists often interview individuals and families about their family history, including who lives in their household and relationships between family members. A genogram is used to visually construct a family tree that records information about family members over the last three generations. A genogram can literally provide a picture of family patterns and help both the family and therapist understand the source of any problems between spouses, parents, and children.

A traditional genogram uses simple shapes to denote family members: circles for females and squares for males. Simple lines are used to show connections between spouses and offspring. A family art therapist may help an individual or a family construct a traditional genogram or may encourage them to make a creative genogram with drawing or collage materials (Figure 9.5). For example, an individual may use personally selected colors and symbols to represent family members and relationships. The purpose is not only to construct a family tree that describes family members and dynamics but also to use materials to create personal symbols of

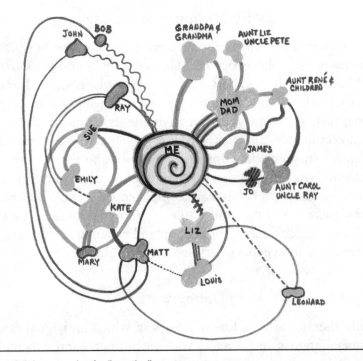

Figure 9.5 An example of a "creative" genogram

parents, siblings, and relatives, which may reveal unconscious beliefs or perceptions.

Art Studio or Open Studio Groups

In contrast to art psychotherapy groups or family art therapy, art studio and open studio groups provide a somewhat different kind of art therapy experience. People who go to art studios are often perceived as artists rather than as patients—artists who are capitalizing on the properties of art making as a process for self-expression, exploration, and healing.

Art therapy has its roots in hospital settings. In the 1940s and 1950s, art therapy was offered to hospitalized patients through therapeutic art studios. These art therapy groups looked very similar to art school studios or adult education classes, and most art therapists who ran them had taught studio classes. Patients who attended these studios could generally come and go (hence, the name open studio) and work in the art therapy studio when it was available and the therapist was present.

The Menninger Clinic in Kansas, mentioned earlier in this book, was one of the first facilities to offer art studios for patients and to employ art as therapy as part of its treatment program. Art was considered an important part of treatment at the clinic. Groups of patients could attend studio arts programs or activity sessions where they were encouraged to make drawings, paintings, sculptures, and crafts as part of their rehabilitation. Art making was believed to be cathartic and to help patients express internal conflicts and achieve insights necessary to their recovery.

Some art therapists feel that the art itself is what is most important and that art making is a process of expressing, discovering, recognizing, and achieving insight without the use of words. Because art therapy involves nonverbal communication through artistic expression, the emphasis is less on traditional talk therapy and more on using the art process to uncover and develop meaning.

While there are many studio-based art therapy programs throughout the United States, there are several that are well known and will give you a good idea of why art studio or open studio groups can be therapeutic.

Raw Art Works

As I discussed previously in Chapter 2, the city of Lynn, Massachusetts, is the backdrop for a unique art therapy program, Raw Art Works (RAW). This community-based program for at-risk children, adolescents, and families uses a studio approach to art therapy that provides inner-city youth with the opportunity to create in a variety of media, including painting, printmaking, collage (as you saw in Figure 2.4 and now in Figure 9.6), sculpture, and filmmaking in the Reel 2 Reel program. The art therapists at RAW use visual arts not only to help individuals express themselves but also as a way to bring together people and facilitate exploration of street violence, substance abuse, and poverty. A young artist at RAW sums up the program and her experience with these observations: "When I step off the elevator into RAW I am thankful to have a place where I can enjoy myself. . . . I can share my feelings and feel accepted."

Raw Art Works has far-reaching effects on its young artists. Many of the youth who originally attended its art programs even-

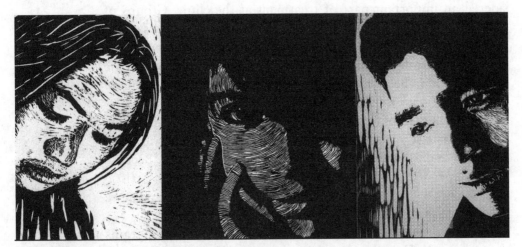

Figure 9.6 Printmaking by participants at the Raw Art Works program in Lynn, Massachusetts
(Reprinted with permission of RAW Arts)

tually went on to become mentors to other teens and younger children, sharing their enthusiasm for creative expression as a way to positively transform their lives. The program has become an alternative to gang involvement for many RAW artists, and among the young mentors, most have stayed in school and 80 percent have applied to college.

Center for Therapy Through the Arts

The Center for Therapy Through the Arts in Cleveland, Ohio, has provided an in-hospital art therapy studio for medically ill and physically disabled people since 1967 and is one of the oldest programs of its kind in the country. Satellite programs also provide unique and innovative community-based art therapy studios for people with neurological disorders, depression, autism, brain injuries, or spinal cord injuries. The organization emphasizes an art-centered approach to therapy and offers an open studio for patient participation, encouraging drop-in visits during studio hours and welcoming family and friends to participate alongside patients or on their own. While the thrust of these group studios is on gaining personal insights, art skills are also taught if patients need help or want to improve abilities for creative expression. Demonstrations from the art therapist, pictures, slides, and other resource materials are often used for motivation. WheelArt—Rolling Toward Wellness, described earlier in the book, is one of the many specialized programs that this center offers.

Art therapist and founder Mary McGraw notes that the Art Studio, a part of the Center for Therapy Through the Arts, emphasizes the uniqueness of each person's creative process. Art therapy sessions focus on two areas within the group setting. Sessions may focus on creative arts experiences that encourage experimentation, learning new information, developing motor or cognitive skills, or enhancing creative thinking through art making. Materials and equipment are accessible, and patients are encouraged to be independent in their choices of media and direction. Or sessions may focus on expressive arts experiences that stimulate the discussion of feelings and promote socialization, communication, and interaction with others. For example, at the end of a group art therapy session, participants may share feelings about the art experience and reflect on each other's artwork, initiating interaction and socialization among group members with the therapist's guidance.

I attended a session at the Art Studio as an outpatient and participated in a small group of adults that met once a week. This particular group was designed around the history of art; each week a different period in art history was used as the theme for the group. The session I attended focused on Egyptian art, and the art therapist shared some examples of paintings, sculptures, wall reliefs, and architecture from that period. After a brief lecture and discussion, we were assigned to create an image of a burial mask similar to the ones used on the pharaohs of ancient Egypt (Figure 9.7). Because the group was held in an art studio setting where drawing, painting, and collage materials were available, we could choose any material to make the mask image. We each worked for more than an hour on our individual images and then were asked to display them on a wall for group feedback and discussion. With the art therapist's guidance, we each described our images and reflected on our process of making the masks.

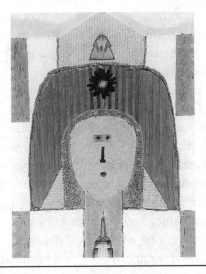

Figure 9.7 The author's Egyptian mask made at the Art Studio at the Cleveland Metropolitan Hospital art therapy program

Art therapy groups at the Art Studio have many different themes and purposes. The outpatient group I attended had several goals. First, it was psychoeducational; that is, not only was it therapeutic, but participants also learned something about art history and how to use art materials. Second, self-expression and creativity were emphasized in the open studio atmosphere. With the help of the art therapist, group members made choices about materials, design, and elements to include in their images. Finally, group interaction was encouraged during the session and in the discussion period at the end. Each person had the chance to share information about his or her image and to respond to the images that others had created.

The Art Studio emphasizes some of the important elements of studio art therapy groups. Working in a studio with other people has elements of collaboration, even when you're working on your own piece. It is impossible not to interact with others and their art expressions. Social support from other artists is central to both the Art Studio and other Center for Therapy Through the Arts programs, affirming the healing potential of group work and creativity to make positive changes in people's physical and emotional lives.

The Open Studio Project

The Open Studio Project (OSP), now located in Evanston, Illinois, began in Chicago in 1991 with the intention to make art and be of service to others. Its philosophy underscores respect for individual creativity and the belief that through creativity, personal meaning can be found and health and wholeness are promoted. The original founders of the OSP—art therapists Pat Allen, Deborah Gadiel, and Dayna Block—created the program based on their belief that art transcends distinctions of age, class, gender, and background. At the OSP, art therapists serve as models and guides by making art alongside participants.

People from all walks of life attend the OSP's workshops and one-week intensives. Open studios are available to patients from hospitals and community agencies, and businesses are encouraged to use the OSP as a place for employees to maintain health and well-being through creative experiences with art making. Mentorship programs allow OSP participants to use art for personal growth in a long-term setting. There are also weekly opportunities to drop in and make art at the studio.

In programs like the OSP, there are opportunities to share one's work, to have others view what one has created, and to discover how art expression can be personally beneficial to health and well-being. I attended a workshop at the original OSP and participated in drop-in time, during which I worked with the rich variety of materials available to participants. There were lots of opportunities to interact with other artists, as well as to work on my own images and process. Programs like the OSP emphasize the principle that art making on its own is essentially a healing process and that an art studio with working artists supports this process.

The Creative Growth Art Center

The Creative Growth Art Center in Oakland, California, directed for more than twenty years by artist–art therapist Irene Ward Brydon, is a nonprofit visual arts organization that provides a studio space in which disabled adults can make art. Any adult who is physically, mentally, or emotionally disabled and interested in art may attend the program. It is not a treatment center, but it provides an enriching environment for creativity through visual arts that benefit participants in many ways.

At Creative Growth, participants are defined as artists rather than clients or patients. Evidence of artistic talent is not necessary, and most participants in the program have not previously attended art classes or been involved with art in any way before coming to the center. The studio program offers more than sixty classes weekly and provides opportunities for painting, drawing, sculpting, ceramics, printmaking, and other art experiences. There are special tools and equipment for those with physical disabilities, as well as a special art studio for participants who are particularly gifted and have the potential to become partially or completely self-supporting through their art.

Creative Growth has a gallery for exhibits of participants' work. It is the first studio of its kind in the United States whose primary mission is to show the art of people with disabilities. Some Creative Growth attendees have become renowned artists in their own right.

One such person is Dwight Mackintosh, who has received international attention for his art. Mackintosh, called "the boy who time forgot," spent fifty-six years of his life in state institutions until, at age seventy-two, he was brought by his brother Earl to the Creative Growth Art Center. While at the center, he has made numerous drawings with a distinctive style, which consists of wavy lines that resemble secret writing or elaborate scribbles. His images often contain people, motor vehicles (generally buses), and buildings, perhaps memories of his many years in institutions. His work is visually powerful, reflecting a world that he is unable to convey except through images (Figure 9.8).

Mackintosh and others who attend programs like Creative Growth demonstrate that even severe disabilities do not necessarily interfere with creativity. By traditional measures of intelligence, Mackintosh is categorized as mildly retarded, but his art shows undeniable talent and skill. All of the participants who come to the center have found that creative activity in the form of art has in some way contributed to their sense of well-being and health. Centers such as Creative Growth have demonstrated that art can reclaim many individuals who have been labeled hopeless cases.

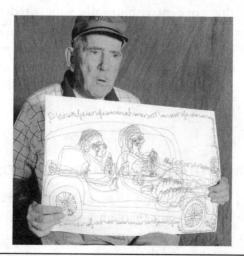

Figure 9.8 Dwight Mackintosh, artist at the Creative Growth Art Center in Oakland, California   *(Reprinted with permission of the Creative Growth Art Center; photograph by Leon Borensztein)*

OFFCenter: Creating Community and Economic Development

OFFCenter Community Arts Project in Albuquerque, New Mexico, is a public program that uses art to build community and to increase self-esteem, self-sufficiency, and hope among homeless individuals and families. The center, located in an urban area, consists of a large studio space where anyone can drop in and make art, including painting, printmaking, mixed media, sculpture, and photography (Figure 9.9).

Since it opened, OFFCenter has been visited by hundreds of people each year. There is a core of regulars, and other people may come to the center to buy art in the studio sales shop. OFFCenter sponsors a number of gallery shows, traveling shows, and collaborative exhibits; it also provides a forum for emerging artists to discuss their creative process and artworks. All ages are welcome, and children are particularly encouraged to attend and make art in a special program designed for participation with family members.

Art therapist and artist Janis Timm-Bottos facilitates the practical workings of OFFCenter. She believes that one of the purposes of the OFFCenter project is to help people value and respect diversity. Since the participants at OFFCenter come from a variety of backgrounds, this concept is naturally supported by the studio atmosphere, where everyone is equal. Timm-Bottos's approach to art therapy is based in the power of community as an agent of change and health. Through interacting with others and sharing art making, people who attend OFFCenter are naturally validated for their creativity.

A Final Word About Drawing Together

Unfortunately, it is not possible to give you an experience of working in an art therapy group through a set of exercises. To understand what it is like to work in a group, whether it be an art psychotherapy group or a therapeutic art studio, you will have to get the experience firsthand.

Another way to experience group art therapy is to attend an art therapy intensive. Art therapy intensives provide participants with an opportunity to experience art as therapy within the span of a day, a weekend, or several days. The goal is to help people learn more about the creative and therapeutic potentials of art making in their lives. You may want to consult the resources section of this book for places to contact to find out more about art therapy intensives. Many colleges, universities, and art centers offer art therapy intensives.

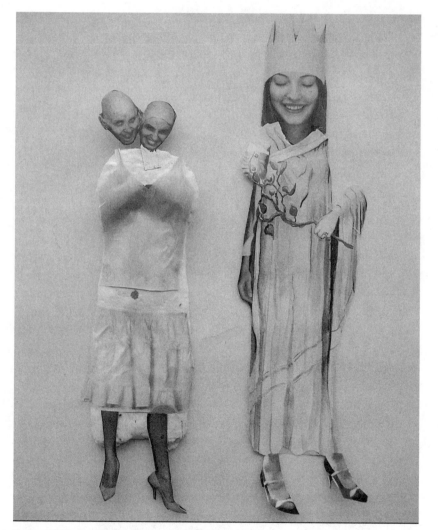

Figure 9.9 Paper dolls by Marisa Faust, OFFCenter Community Arts Project, Albuquerque, New Mexico
(Reprinted with permission of Janis Timm-Bottos, director, OFFCenter)

Art making within a group or studio is different from working alone. If you are interested in deepening your understanding of the healing potentials of art making, it is well worth your time to participate in an art therapy group or an open studio program. Both group art psychotherapy and therapeutic art studios encourage interaction between members and offer a unique way to experience the therapeutic and creative value of art activities.

10

Working with the Art Product: Drawing on Meaning

The image doesn't represent imagination—but it takes imagination to get to know who the image is.

Paolo Knill, Helen Barba, and Margo Fuchs,
Minstrels of the Soul

Art therapists have developed many ways of working with images. Some of their techniques and methods are based in psychology, while others are based in the visual and expressive arts (music, movement, drama, and writing).

The "Talking Cure"

Most art therapists believe it is important to encourage people to talk about their images in some way. Talking about the content of one's images with a therapist not only helps a person to derive meaning from them, but the process of talking is also believed to be healing in and of itself. It is believed that through the "talking cure," upsetting experiences, memories, and feelings can be alleviated and resolved.

The idea of the talking cure came about more than a hundred years ago and has been one of the mainstays of verbal therapy. Joseph Breuer, a physician in the late nineteenth century, is thought to have been one of the first to explore the talking cure during his work with hypnosis. One of his most important cases was with a young woman referred to as Anna O., who suffered from a variety of emotional problems and psychosomatic symptoms. Breuer requested that Anna O. talk about her early experiences and her symptoms while under hypnosis. He conjectured that through talking about her traumas, Anna O. began to recover and was eventually cured of her problems.

Freud was intrigued by Breuer's reports and success. Although Freud used hypnosis with his patients, he also found that he could achieve similar success without hypnosis through merely having his patients talk about their feelings and thoughts. Both Freud and Breuer came to believe that the talking cure allowed people to release emotions that they were suppressing.

There is disagreement about how talking helps to alleviate trauma and encourage emotional recovery. Some believe that talking about emotionally distressing experiences is valuable because it encourages catharsis, allowing a person to express conflicts and feelings. Others feel that talking helps a person gain insight into his or her problems, identifying the source of the difficulty and possible ways to mitigate it. Even Freud eventually came to the conclusion that more than catharsis was necessary to achieve results through talking. Most therapists today believe that it is important for people to gain some insight as to the cause and effect of trauma they have experienced. Through talking about upsetting experiences and conflicts with a therapist, a person comes to understand the origin and consequences of distressing emotions and, as a result, is better able to deal with them.

The exact nature of how the talking cure works in conjunction with art therapy is still debatable and is explained differently by different therapists. Most art therapists seem to agree that some form of talking about art expressions is important and beneficial. Some integrate theories and methods that are common to verbal therapies in their work with people and their art expressions. Art therapy approaches that are strongly influenced by Freud and his followers are aimed at achieving insight both through talking and through receiving comments from the therapist. Other approaches emphasize the art therapist's acceptance, receptive listening, and respect for people's creative abilities as important aspects of talking about art expressions. Most therapists believe that people are better able to arrive at meanings for their images when they talk about them with a professional who can guide their process of discovery.

The Therapeutic Alliance

Art therapy, like other forms of therapy, is based on the therapeutic alliance. This alliance involves trust between the therapist and the person in therapy and a commitment on the part of both to achieving therapeutic goals. Therapists since Freud's time have believed that this relationship is critical in helping people confront painful feelings and events in their lives, achieve positive change, and resolve conflicts.

Art therapy presents a somewhat unique therapeutic alliance for several reasons. In art therapy, the therapist often assumes a more active role in the process because he or she may be teaching the person some art skills or demonstrating how to use materials. There is naturally more physical activity in art therapy as opposed to strictly verbal therapy because art making is involved. Also, in art therapy, personal expression is shared through some form of art rather than solely through words. The art expression becomes part of the interaction; in other words, the person interacts not only with the therapist but also with the art-making process and the art product.

In any type of therapy, the therapeutic fit between the therapist and person seeking therapy is key to the success of the treatment. In art therapy, it is important that the therapist's views of art making and the person's preferences match. For example, some therapists focus more on talking about images than on making them. Other therapists may focus more on the art process, encouraging the person to have more in-depth experiences with art materials and techniques. Many therapists combine approaches in their work with people or use different approaches depending on the person, the goals of therapy, and the context. The success of the therapeutic alliance in art therapy depends on how well the therapist's way of working meets the person's needs and goals for art making as therapy.

Theoretical orientation is also part of the art therapy relationship, and therapists use a variety of philosophies and techniques depending on their training and preferences. The following approaches are some of the more common ones that art therapists may use to help people work with their art expressions, approaches that generally include both talking and art making.

Free Association and Interpretation

Art therapy has been greatly influenced by the work and ideas of Margaret Naumburg, who has been mentioned throughout this book for her role in developing the field of art therapy. Naumburg was one of the first people in the United States to undergo psychoanalysis. She began working as an art therapist when Freudian psychology was popular, and she promoted the importance of making the unconscious conscious. Though she incorporated Jung's ideas and other theories into her philosophy, Freudian psychology had a major influence on her work as an art therapist. As a result, Naumburg emphasized releasing unconscious material through art expression and modeled her approach on that of psychoanalysis, particularly the technique of free association.

Naumburg, like many art therapists, thought that the real meaning of art expressions came only from the people who made them. She believed that art has projective qualities; that is, the job of the therapist is to help a person find meaning for his or her images through spontaneously assigning meaning to content. Naumburg saw art as symbolic speech, a starting place for free expression, to be followed by verbal associations with the image. The therapist and the patient then work together toward understanding the image, drawing inferences about how its content may relate to the person's life.

An important part of this approach is the concept of transference, the projection of the person's unresolved feelings, perceptions, and ideas onto the therapist. Transference refers to the way that person unconsciously responds to the therapist as if responding to a significant individual in the person's past. Conflicts from previous relationships, such as with a parent, may begin to surface or may be reflected in the art created in therapy. For example, a person may react to the therapist as an authority figure or a parent, behaving or communicating unresolved issues or wishes through art or speech. The person may respond negatively to the therapist as if to a strict and unloving parental figure, or positively, perhaps seeking the therapist's approval and acceptance. A person may also transfer or project feelings, thoughts, fantasies, and conflicts onto art images.

The therapist uses the person's transference to understand his or her beliefs and behaviors, particularly any unsettled conflicts or feelings. The therapist may encourage the person to explore and work through transference through a variety of techniques, including free association and interpretation. Free association, or saying whatever comes to mind, was mentioned earlier in this book and is essentially a form of spontaneous expression. The therapist may invite the person to free associate feelings, fantasies, and perceptions about the images created. In listening to the person's free associations, the therapist may hear hidden meanings and recognize unconscious material emerging in the person's art expressions.

In a psychoanalytic approach to art therapy, the therapist tries to help the person understand emotional problems, inner conflicts, or negative behaviors through clarifying, questioning, or confronting. Interpretation can also be an important part of the process. In the case of art therapy, a therapist may help a person to make connections between his or her images and perceptions, feelings, or behaviors in his or her life. The underlying purpose is to assist the person in gaining insight into the hidden meaning and relevance of behavior and emotions.

Active Imagination

Many therapists use a method of working with images proposed by Jung called active imagination. Jung realized through his own experiences with mental images that one had to directly enter into them to understand them. He simply defined active imagination as "a sequence of fantasies produced by deliberate concentration" on an image. Jung also referred to active imagination as "dreaming the dream onward," a way of freely associating from the original image experienced in a dream to other images, thoughts, and feelings as they arise. This technique can also be used with drawings, paintings, and other art images, helping a person generate a story from his or her art. The use of active imagination with images in art therapy is also referred to as image dialogue because it follows picture making, as opposed to dreams, and may be used to generate another series of images.

The associations that one makes with a drawing or painting through active imagination are spontaneous and uncensored and reflect life experiences and perceptions, environmental influences, and universal symbols. In exploring your images through active imagination, you may discover personal, cultural, and universal associations. Active imagination was thought by Jung to tap the universal world of myth and heritage—the collective unconscious—and reveal archetypes, the contents of the collective unconscious.

During the process of active imagination, a therapist may work with the person to deepen his or her understanding of elements of the collective unconscious, particularly the persona, the anima and animus, and the shadow. The persona is essentially the mask or public face we wear to protect ourselves. The anima and animus represent aspects of femininity and masculinity that are believed to exist in both sexes. Jung observed that it is important to recognize these opposite parts of the self in order to integrate and balance them. The shadow represents the dark side of the self—thoughts, feelings, and actions that we find reproachable in others. The shadow is generally the same sex as the individual and may take the form of a threatening, evil, or criminal figure or may simply have characteristics of someone we dislike in day-to-day life. Jung believed that a shadow exists in all of us and that through imagery found in dreams or art, we can express and acknowledge this dark side.

The goal of active imagination is to help you explore yourself through metaphor and to develop a spontaneous, personal narrative to enhance understanding, insight, and growth. It is a very powerful way of working with images and is a skill that often takes time to develop, even with the help of a therapist. I have found that in working with my own images and helping others to use active imagination in processing their own art, associations and stories seem to come in stages. You may have to return to the image at a later time and continue the process. It underscores that fully understanding images takes time, that images have many meanings, and that interpretation is shaped by personal, cultural, and universal dimensions.

Gestalt Techniques

Gestalt therapy is most often associated with Fritz Perls, who practiced at the Esalen Institute in California in the 1960s. Gestalt therapy grew out of Gestalt psychology, which emerged in the early 1900s and emphasized understanding how people perceive and learn. The word *gestalt* is German and roughly means "form, pattern, structure, or configuration." Gestalt psychologists studied, among other things, how we naturally tend to visually perceive parts to make a whole. For example, when we look at a form that is almost a circle, we tend to see a whole circle, visually completing the shape and closure of that form.

Gestalt therapists based their practice on some of the theories of Gestalt psychology, adapting them to work with people in therapeutic settings. The word *gestalt* emphasizes understanding an individual's personality as a totality of many parts and a person's experience of being in the world—in other words, the whole picture.

While psychoanalytic approaches to therapy generally focus on an examination of how the past affects the present, Gestalt therapy is more interested in the here and now. The therapist helps people become aware of what events, experiences, or perceptions in the present are creating problems for them. This process is often referred to as taking care of unfinished business. In Gestalt approaches, personal responsibility is stressed, and individuals are encouraged to make their own interpretations. Transference is not encouraged and is seen as an avoidance of a person-to-person relationship between the therapist and client.

Art therapist Janie Rhyne is best known for Gestalt approaches to art therapy and refers to them as "Gestalt art experiences." A therapist who uses Gestalt approaches in art therapy may use the art products as a reference and catalyst for discussion. The elements of the art product may be viewed as a whole, and additional techniques—such as movement, dramatic enactment, or sound—may be used to help the individual arrive at meaning. For example, the person may be encouraged to create a movement, dance, or sound that expresses the colors, lines, and shapes of the art expression. In a group, the person might be asked to direct others to enact the elements of the art piece. The therapist might say, "Use the people in this group to be your shapes, colors, and lines, and ask them to enact the sounds or movement you choose to represent the art expression." The goal is to help the person become more conscious of all his or her senses, using them to increase self-awareness.

Because Gestalt art approaches emphasize a holistic view, they are often used to broaden people's understanding of how they function within groups and to help individuals discover new insights about themselves through group activities. The therapist is the leader of the group as well as part of the group. In a Gestalt art therapy group, a person may learn through art activities to develop interpersonal skills. For example, the group may be asked to create a drawing depicting what they would need to coexist on an island. Through the activity and group discussion after the art experience, participants may learn new communication skills, how they negotiate and interact with others, and how they feel about coexisting within a group.

Lastly, a therapist using a Gestalt approach may ask you to talk from art expressions rather than talk about them. For example, you may be asked to identify with your images by looking at your work and describing it through phrases such as "I am" or "I feel." In other words, instead of saying that your painting has a lot of red circles in it, you might say, "I am many red circles, and I feel crowded, happy, passionate, and playful," personifying elements in your artwork and using them to describe your own experiences and perceptions. The emphasis in a Gestalt art therapy process is on developing and expressing your own meaning for images, defined from your own perspective and from the here and now.

Person-Centered Approaches

The person-centered, or client-centered, approach to counseling was developed by well-known humanistic psychologist Carl Rogers. Rogers felt that the role of the therapist was to be open, empathetic, honest, and caring and to facilitate the growth of the individual through therapy. He believed that the best way to understand people is from people themselves and their own internal frames of reference.

A person-centered philosophy to expressive arts therapy has been formulated by Natalie Rogers; it is based on the theories and methods of her father, Carl. Through what Natalie Rogers terms the "creative connection" between all the arts, therapy emphasizes self-actualization and finding one's own meaning through self-expression. She believes that through creative expression people learn how to become authentic, self-actualized, and connected with their true purpose in life. While Natalie Rogers's approach utilizes all the arts (art, music, movement, and drama), an art therapist may use a person-centered approach through offering art experiences with the purpose of enhancing creative potential and self-understanding. Using art as a modality for personal growth and insight is based on the belief that the creative process is healing and that all people have the innate ability to be creative.

There are no specific methods in the person-centered approach. The techniques are the therapist's attitudes of empathetic understanding, caring, respect, acceptance, and reflection, responses that encourage clients to make positive choices and decisions. Nondirective approaches to art making (experiences that involve free choice of subject matter) are offered, to encourage the use of personal creativity to explore the self. Empowerment through art is central to the therapeutic process in the person-centered approach, and exploring one's creative potential is believed to be the key to personal transformation.

Systems Theory Approaches

Family art therapy was described in Chapter 9 as a way of working with individuals, couples, or families. Most family art therapy uses systems theory to assess communication patterns within the person's family. Systems theory is based on the philosophy that individuals are best understood through appraising the interactions within an entire family. In this approach, a person's emotional problems are viewed as an expression of a larger problem within the person's family. For example, the case of the little girl who developed an ulcer due to stress within her family (described in Chapter 8) could easily be understood from systems theory. From this perspective, the girl's ulcer could represent an expressed pain that pervaded the entire family, caused by unresolved distress in the entire system. A therapist working from a systems perspective might use art activities with the whole family to increase communication and resolve problems, or he or she might use art with the girl to explore her perceptions of her parents and siblings.

Because a systems theory approach emphasizes relationships between family members, an art therapist may use a variety of techniques that focus on identifying and understanding family dynamics. The therapist might ask a client to make a genogram (see Chapter 9) that shows how the person views his or her family of origin and what interactive patterns are present. Or the therapist might request that a family work together to make a collage or work in pairs on a drawing to identify communication patterns and behaviors. Art activities may also be used to help family members learn to solve problems creatively, and experientials may be designed to achieve specific goals in improving interpersonal skills between family members.

Creative Arts in Counseling

Many art therapists are also mental health counselors, and a number of mental health counselors, social workers, marriage and family therapists, and psychologists use art therapy along with verbal counseling in their work. Creative arts are often used in counseling in conjunction with a specific counseling approach to enhance therapy, move the individual to action, express thoughts, practice behaviors, and help the client to examine options.

Solution-focused counseling is one approach that is often successfully combined with visual arts. Drawing, collage, or other activities are used to help individuals explore solutions to problems rather than search for explanations for why the problem occurred. The goal is to set an expectation for change and to encourage individuals to actively participate in creating changes in themselves and in their lives. For example, the solution-focused counselor may ask individuals who are depressed to imagine a time when they were not depressed and draw an image of what that time would look like. Or the counselor might request that they imagine what their lives would look like if they awoke one day and were symptom free (Figure 10.1). This "miracle question" helps a client to speculate what life would be like when the problem brought to counseling is actually solved by using creative expression as the catalyst.

Narrative strategies are also used in creative arts and counseling. The goal of narrative therapy is to help the client understand personal problems and conflicts by externalizing them and to separate the person from his or her problems. In traditional narrative therapy, individuals externalize their problems through telling their stories and exploring new outcomes for their stories with the help

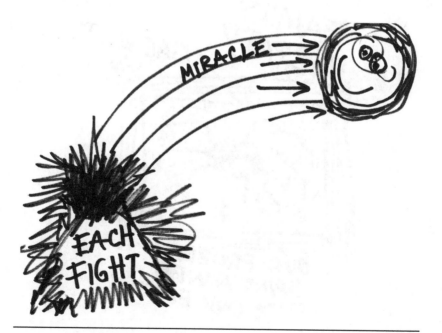

Figure 10.1 A drawing of what a "miracle" would look like

of the counselor. In creative arts and counseling, art expression becomes a form of externalization, helping the problem to become visible. For example, in a family therapy session, one participant depicted the dominant problem in her family as a "web over our family" (Figure 10.2). When asked what she could do to change this situation through adding something to the drawing, she placed a box around the web, saying that family therapy could help "cage it in." In this case, drawing a solution to changing the family problem and working with the counselor to create a new story for overcoming her emotional difficulties helped her to imagine a new scenario and outcome.

Most uses of creative arts in counseling support the idea that the counselor and client are partners and collaborators in problem solving. These approaches capitalize on the potential of art expression to make internal thoughts, feelings, and solutions visible and

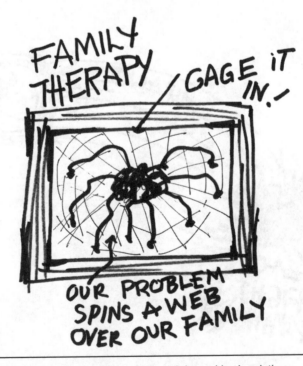

Figure 10.2 A drawing of a family's problem and the problem's solution

tangible, giving the person the ability to externalize, reframe, and "restory" the problem or conflict.

"Third-Hand" Approaches

Art therapist Edith Kramer emphasized the importance of helping people in art therapy achieve artistic expression. She suggested that it is important to intervene during the art-making process to help the person improve on his or her expression without distorting the image or the person's original intent. Kramer referred to this as "using the art therapist's third hand." This approach stresses art as therapy, in which the process of making art is considered important.

For example, the therapist might start a drawing for the child to finish or save a child's clay figure from falling apart by reinforcing the legs. In some situations, I have used my own art making to develop a relationship with an adult or a child. For example, in working with a child who would not talk, I drew portraits of the child to engage her interest in establishing a relationship with me. As she began to trust me, she was able to pick up a crayon and make a joint drawing with me. Eventually, she was able to draw on her own and to choose materials and themes for her own creations.

Sometimes I am asked to make third-hand interventions by people who need help with drawing or painting because of physical limitations. Brent, a thirty-six-year-old man with cancer, had lost most of the sensitivity in his hands as a result of chemotherapy. Although he could not use his hands comfortably, Brent still enjoyed making collages. He could choose colors and images but often did not have enough dexterity to cut and glue the pieces. I served as the third hand in cutting and gluing, while Brent made all the decisions about images and composition. Following his instructions, I prepared, placed, and secured the images in arrangements he created.

Some therapists work on art right alongside their patients. While this is more likely in group sessions, some therapists paint or draw during individual sessions, too. Many therapists believe this practice models creative behavior and establishes an environment in which positive change and growth can take place.

Integrative Arts Therapies, or Expressive Therapy Approaches

While most ways of working with art images involve talking, some methods focus more heavily on the use of the arts themselves to explore meaning. Integrative approaches, also known as expressive therapies, rely on the arts as a way to express and deepen understanding of one's imagery. Expressive therapy is recognized as a therapeutic method that includes a variety of modalities for self-expression—art, music, movement, drama, play, and writing. In other words, rather than asking you to explain the contents of an image, a therapist using an integrative arts therapy or expressive therapy approach might encourage you to respond to it through other art forms. Expressive therapists Paolo Knill, Helen Barba, and Margo Fuchs, in *Minstrels of the Soul*, describe dreams as an example of the intermodal qualities of imagination: "Consider dreams, where the soul speaks through imagination. We may sense the movement of swimming or hear a voice or speak words; we may experience the act of killing or see a beautiful visual image of a city, or listen to the sound and rhythm of music."

In an integrative arts therapy session, you might be asked to create a sound to describe a color or form in a drawing or painting. Or you might be asked to use movement to enact an emotion or experience, then to create a sound or music to describe the feeling, and then perhaps to paint an image of that experience using lines and shapes that reflect the rhythm and movement. Expressive therapists believe that an integrative approach may bring increased understanding and a deeper experience because you use a variety of sensory methods of self-expression for personal exploration.

Writing and Poetry

Creative writing is one of the more popular integrative approaches. For this reason, it deserves a more in-depth discussion. James Pennebaker, who has researched the role of writing in health and well-being, has established that writing about painful experiences is key to successful recovery, both physically and emotionally. Writing about traumatic events in particular can be health giving and anxiety reducing, and studies indicate that it is helpful in trauma recovery and in the reduction of symptoms of arthritis.

Creative writing, in the form of prose or poetry, deepens the experience of image making, and, for some people, it stimulates creative potential in a way that art cannot. Richard, a young man with AIDS who came to my private practice for several years, used poetry as a way to describe and understand his art expressions and his experience of life-threatening illness. Because of his illness, Richard had difficulty manipulating art materials, so instead of drawing or painting, he worked collage. Because Richard enjoyed writing poetry, I asked him to try writing poems about some of the images he selected for his collages, to further explore their meaning in a creative way.

One particular image Richard felt drawn to was a photograph of a toy soldier, dressed for combat and holding binoculars up to his eyes. The soldier raised one hand as if to signal or wave to someone he saw in the distance. Richard used this image as the centerpiece of a small collage he made one day during an art therapy session. In response to the image, he wrote the following poem between sessions:

What am I looking at
Who do I see
A helmet on my head
Fatigues to each knee

Belts of ammunition
Adorn my military gear
Camouflage and olive drab
Could be "IN" this year

A funny garb of armor
Beetle Bailey and the Sarge
Characters from comic books
I'll take an extra large

A stealthful watch, a reconnaissance
I make through inquisitive eyes
While insects forage below me
Blue birds tango across the skies

Something in the distance
Binoculars aid my sight
Does life exist on the planet Mars
Is there a reason for cellulite

My intellect asks many questions
Nagging headaches do ensue
But aspirin are not needed
Only this Shaman's old voodoo

Listening with intensity
A child's laughter does resound
A familiar voice once silenced
Now calls from "lost and found"

I raise my hand with confidence
To greet the vast unknown
Thoughts of Spielberg and E.T.
And me without a phone

No apparent boundaries
Many paths are undefined
My inner guides and trusted scout
Say seek and ye shall find

Stars spiral in a celestial oasis
Like munchkins in the land of Oz
The transcendence of spirit through the color of light
Leads us onward in reverent cause

My battle scars are many
Over lifetimes expansive and deep
Angelic choirs sing sweet lullabies
Mr. Sandman brings enchanted sleep

Music soothes the savage beast
But what of a lonely heart
Tell me what you're dreamin' of
My soulful counterpart

I imagine your touch in heaven
Your love fills me up so
Caressed by a meadow of poppies
And plumes of indigo

The Wisdom of the Ages
Cascading sands in an hourglass
Fleeting moments and precious memories
I recall while lying in the grass

A destiny awakens
The blessed miracle of birth
Death is a wondrous beginning
Now, Voyager, safe passage from Earth

Richard's sense of humor and skill with words are apparent in this poem. He is obviously a gifted poet, and writing poems and short stories about his collages tapped his personal creativity, helping him cope with his illness and alleviating some of the depression he often experienced. However, I find that people do not need to be talented writers to benefit from writing about their images. Writing a few lines, either in the form of a poem or prose, can be helpful in deepening the experience of art making. Like most art therapists, I find that when people share with me their own words about their art, my understanding of their experiences is also expanded, and I am better able to guide the art therapy process.

Art and Play

In working with children, art therapy is often combined with play therapy techniques. Play therapy includes the use of art activities, therapeutic toys, games, puppets, and other props to help children; it has also been applied to work with adults and even families. Very young children benefit from art and play therapy because they often cannot adequately express their thoughts and feelings with words alone.

For Marie, a seven-year-old girl who had been sexually abused, art and play provided a window to her depression and recurrent nightmares. She had been abused several times by a trusted family member, who threatened her into silence. Marie used painting to convey what she could not say out loud, often depicting herself as a frightened little girl with no one to help her (Figure 10.3).

As she became less anxious and afraid during the course of therapy, she began to use play activities to communicate a growing sense of trust and safety. Marie first used a pretend phone in the playroom to communicate with the therapist, indicating her growing trust. Through play with puppets, Marie dramatized scenarios in which adult animals took care of baby animals by providing them with a safe home in which to live and taking care of their needs for

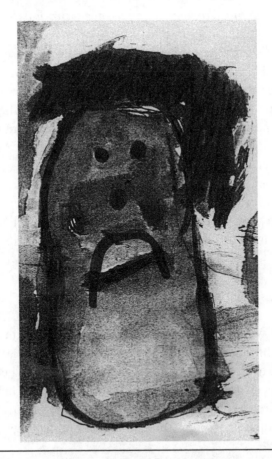

Figure 10.3 Marie's painting of herself as frightened and helpless

food and nurturance. For a plastic figure of a cat, she created a "safe world," in which all of its needs were met. She selected objects in the playroom that represented food, water, a cozy bed, and cat toys for play to make the cat feel more comfortable and protected.

By the end of her therapy, Marie's personality had become more outgoing and confident—reflected in a colorful self-portrait of her with a large smile and outreaching arms. Like many abused children, many months passed before she began to overcome her fears and depression.

The combination of art and play in therapy provides children like Marie with the opportunity to recover from stressful experiences, using a variety of symbols either self-created through art or used as metaphors in the form of toys and props. The universal nature of art and play, activities that most children perceive as nonthreatening and familiar, when used together in treatment, helped Marie express her experiences as well as to play out new possibilities during the course of her recovery.

Integrative, or Eclectic, Approaches to Art Therapy

Although some art therapists use one general philosophy to guide their work with people, many use a combination of the techniques mentioned in this chapter. This practice of using several approaches is often referred to as eclectic, but I prefer to call it integrative because approaches are usually combined and synthesized to provide the most appropriate and best possible therapeutic experience for the person or group.

For example, in my work with children, I often use a third-hand approach as well as expressive therapy techniques, because children enjoy using their bodies to move or make rhythms and sounds to express themselves. In working with trauma survivors, I may ask them to write about their art expressions, using the journal exercises described throughout this book to help them express emotional distress; I may also use family art therapy techniques to help them explore relationships. I may use some Gestalt techniques and a systems approach to help a family solve a problem, and with a group of cancer survivors I might use active imagination and witnessing as a way of sharing their art with each other. Most therapists choose approaches based not only on their personal philosophy but also on what an individual or a group needs.

Projective Drawings and Art-Based Assessments

Because art is a powerful way of understanding personality, emotions, and perceptions, it is used by some therapists as a form of assessment. As mentioned early in this book, psychiatrists since the early 1900s have been interested in how drawings and other art expressions could be useful in understanding personality, particularly in diagnosing mental illness. Jung saw the potential of art to express symbols from the unconscious, but he did not propose a specific way of interpreting its content. Freud was more closely associated with interpretation of dreams and images. In 1913 Freud spent several weeks drawing and studying Michelangelo's statue of Moses. He then wrote an extensive interpretation of the sculpture, noting symbolic content of the work and aspects that he believed reflected the artist's personality. Freud's experience, however, demonstrates that to understand an image one must spend a long time studying it.

During the 1940s and 1950s, the use of drawings to understand personality became popular and helped psychologists and others to further their understanding of personality, behavior, and development. Today, art therapists, psychologists, and other therapists use drawings for the purpose of assessment and evaluation of mental disorders and emotional problems. This specialized use of drawings involves training and understanding of the complexities of art expressions and the people who make them.

Therapists use several common projective drawing techniques to further their understanding of personality, behavior, and development. Projective drawing tasks usually involve drawing simple themes, such as a house, a tree, and a human figure, or one's family. These techniques may be employed as part of a psychological assessment, or they may be used when therapists want to understand particular aspects of an individual. Some projective techniques involve both drawing and answering a series of questions after completing the drawing. For example, the House-Tree-Person (HTP) drawing includes a postdrawing interview in which the therapist may ask the person about various elements in the drawings, such as: How old is the person in the drawing? Is that a man or a woman? What is he or she doing? Is the tree alone or in a group of trees? What is the house made of? What is the weather in this picture (what time of day, sky, temperature)? The answers to these and other questions are thought to provide information on personality by allowing you to project and convey beliefs about your drawings.

More recently, several methods of evaluating drawings have been developed. Following are descriptions of some of the more widely used drawing evaluation tasks in the field of art therapy.

The Diagnostic Drawing Series (DDS) is not a projective drawing test per se but rather a series of drawing activities designed to provide information on personality, emotional disorders, trauma, and other conditions. The DDS requires three drawings on 18 × 24 inch paper with chalk pastels and asks the participant to do the following:

1. Make a picture using these materials.
2. Draw a tree.
3. Using lines, shapes, and colors, make a picture of how you are feeling.

The drawings are evaluated for their structural qualities, color, and content.

The Silver Drawing Test (SDT) uses a set of "stimulus drawings," which include line drawings of people, animals, places, and objects (Figure 10.4). Some of the pictures are explicit and others are ambiguous to encourage the individual to make personal associations with them. The SDT has two parts. First, the person selects two stimulus images and makes a drawing including both, imagining that something is happening between the two images chosen. If desired, the person may add other features or objects. Then the per-

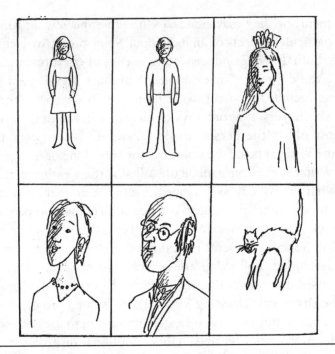

Figure 10.4 An example of drawings used in the Silver Drawing Test
(Reprinted from Three Art Assessments *© 2002 Rawley Silver, with permission of Routledge/ Taylor & Francis Group, LLC)*

son is asked to provide a title, write a short story about the picture, and share the story and its meaning with the therapist (Figure 10.5).

The Formal Elements Art Therapy Scale (FEATS) is another evaluating tool that is used to quantify variables in drawings, particularly drawings of a "person picking an apple from a tree (PPAT)," a task developed by Viktor Lowenfeld, well known for his contributions to understanding children's art. The FEATS can be used to measure characteristics such as composition, line quality, color, and logic of the PPAT and, on a limited basis, other drawings. It has been widely employed to evaluate the structural characteristics and content of drawings by psychiatric patients as well as other individuals. Rather than identify or diagnose psychiatric disorders, the objective of the FEATS tool is to compare possible changes in psychological states during the course of treatment or therapy.

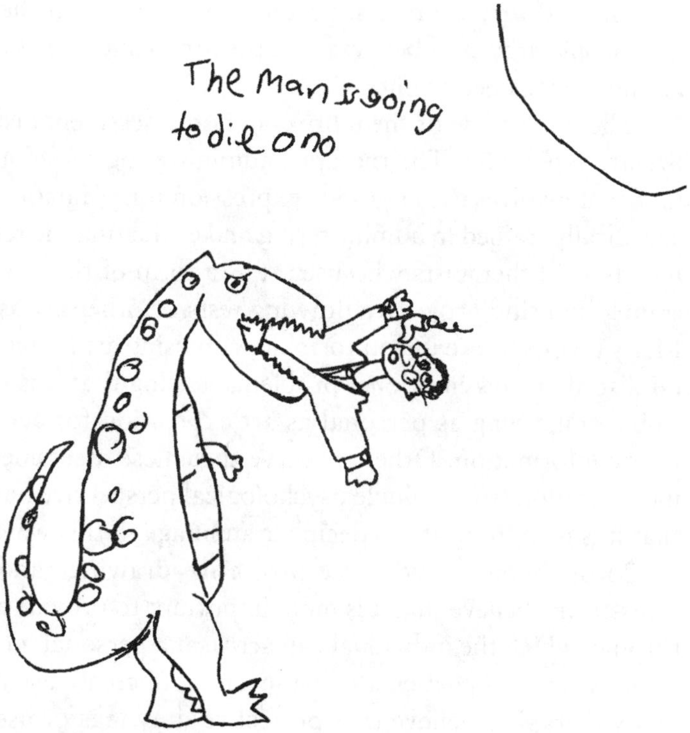

Figure 10.5 *The man is going to die o no*, an example of part of a Silver Drawing Test, by Carl, age twelve   *(Reprinted from* Aggression and Depression Assessed Through Art *© 2005 Rawley Silver, editor, with permission of Routledge/Taylor & Francis Group, LLC)*

As discussed in Chapter 6, mandala drawings have also been used as indicators of personality. In the Mandala Assessment Research Instrument (MARI) card test, a person is asked to select from a set of mandala design cards a series of mandala images and then to choose a color for each design from a set of colored cards. The person is then asked to draw two mandalas—one on white paper and one on black paper—using oil pastels. Next, the person is asked to provide feedback on the experience, which will reveal additional information on personal meaning and content. The MARI card test is designed to assess an individual's present state and is thought to give clues to various psychological processes at work. Its interpretation is based on the theories of Joan Kellogg, who sees recurring images, patterns, and shapes in the mandalas that people draw and believes that the forms and colors are clues to an individual's personality.

These are a few of the more common assessment tasks that utilize art expression. The therapist administering these or any other task that involves the use of art expression for evaluation should be specifically trained in administering and evaluating the results of the test. Not all therapists who use art as a form of therapy have been trained in using projective drawing tests or other art assessments. Many therapists are uncomfortable with using art to diagnose mental disorders and emotional problems, feeling that it is not feasible to use something as personal as art expression for accurate diagnostic information. Others observe that these assessments rely on interpretation from a single psychological perspective or theory and that it is inappropriate to decipher an image in this way.

Most therapists who use projective drawings and art-based assessments believe that it is more important to provide experiences through which the individual can arrive at a personal interpretation of drawings and participate in a meaningful creative activity. Also, many therapists believe that projective drawings or assigned subjects are less useful because they limit what the person will express. "Draw whatever you want" may provide a broader opportunity for the person to reflect current issues or feelings.

Working on Your Own

Finally, there are some simple questions that you can ask yourself about your work and art activities to continue your exploration and to deepen your experience, in lieu of working with a therapist. While this is not a substitute for the therapeutic interaction that is part of art therapy, it will help you begin to understand your own images.

What Feeling Does the Image Communicate?

When you look at the drawing, painting, or other art expression, a feeling is always conveyed. Rather than determining or assigning a meaning, try to look at the image for its emotional quality. What are your initial impressions? Is the image happy, angry, sad, anxious, and so on? Or does it have many different feelings expressed through color, line, and form? How do you use color, line, and form to express emotion?

If the Image Could Talk to You, What Would It Say?

Pretend that you can animate the image you have created. Look at various parts of your image and give each a voice. For example, if there is a blue square in the image, what would that blue square say? Or if you selected an image of a tree from a magazine for a collage, what would that tree say? Try answering these questions in the first person ("I am a tree and I feel . . ."), spontaneously writing down whatever comes to mind.

Amplify a Part of the Image

Look at the image you have created, and select a section of it that interests you or perhaps one that you dislike. Try making another drawing or painting of that section only, enlarging it and adding new details or images that come to mind. Continue this process as long as you wish.

Explore Images with Images

You may also want to try using art as a way to understand and become more aware of your process and images. Try making another image in response to the original one. Continue this process as long as you wish or with as many images as necessary.

What do you do if nothing comes to mind? First, don't worry. It is not necessary to have a meaning for each image right after you create it. I find that some ideas appear soon after the image is completed and many others emerge with time. Don't expect to be able to immediately freely associate, amplify, or understand everything you draw, paint, or construct.

Also, your images will have different meanings as days and weeks pass. Don't think that your task is over once you have defined what an image means in a particular painting or drawing. That meaning may change, or it may provide clues to other works you have created. Keep an open mind, stay free of conclusions, and continue your exploration.

Remember, too, that the processes of drawing, painting, constructing, or building are just as important as finding meaning for your work. You will usually discover that the creative process itself is truly the most healing part of any art therapy experience.

If you are still hungry for information or you want to work with an art therapist, explore an art therapy group, attend a workshop, or deepen your understanding through additional reading, turn to the final section. The resources listed there will increase your knowledge and broaden your experience with art therapy.

Going Further: Drawing on Resources

To FURTHER YOUR knowledge of art therapy, you may want to draw on some of the many available resources. This section provides information on a variety of organizations, websites, journals, and books that can expand your understanding of art therapy and related uses of visual arts for healing. Those who are looking for an art therapist in their area will find a helpful tool in the first section. Readers who wish to know more about what it takes to become an art therapist will find some answers to their questions in the second section.

Finding an Art Therapist

The American Art Therapy Association (AATA) offers a public service, ArtTherapistLocator (arttherapistlocator.org), to help potential clients and related professionals find professional art therapists in their region. This website has searchable features, such as location, specialties, and populations served, as well as links to art therapists' websites. Only art therapists who are professional members of the AATA and have met the educational and postgraduate standards for becoming a professional art therapist can be listed on this site.

How Do I Become an
Art Therapist?

As described in Chapter 10, a variety of workshops and intensives can give you the experience of art therapy. There are also formal art therapy courses available at the undergraduate and graduate levels at colleges and universities across the United States. Undergraduate courses are usually introductory and serve as a foundation for those individuals who want to obtain a graduate degree in art therapy. Opportunities to work under the supervision of an art therapist or to volunteer in an art therapy program are also offered. If you are wondering if you would enjoy working as an art therapist, these courses and experiences are a good place to begin.

While undergraduate art therapy courses have a great deal to offer, a master's degree is regarded as the entry level for professional art therapists. Because art therapists often work in capacities similar to those of master's-level mental health counselors, marriage and family therapists, or social workers, the standards for art therapy training set forth by the AATA require a master's degree and equivalent course work. There are currently more than fifty graduate-level training programs in art therapy at colleges and universities throughout the United States and Canada. Some of these training programs offer a master's degree in art therapy, expressive therapy, or creative arts therapies, while others may offer a degree in counseling with an emphasis in art therapy.

If you plan to undertake graduate-level training in art therapy, it is important to consider what you want from an educational program. For example, if you plan to work in clinical settings, such as hospitals or psychiatric facilities, or as a private or an independent practitioner, you may need a degree in counseling with an emphasis in art therapy. This type of degree will help you become eligible to be licensed as a mental health counselor in addition to obtaining a credential as a professional art therapist. If you plan to work in a particular state after graduation, check the state laws and regulations regarding mental health counseling licenses and art therapy. Some state licensure boards accept art therapy degrees as equivalent to counseling degrees. Others, however, require that one's degree title include the word *counseling*.

Before you invest your time in a training program, determine whether you need a specific degree title to meet your eventual career goals after graduation, especially if your goals include licensure for reimbursement by insurance companies and health care plans. The academic adviser, program director, or career counselor at the college or university you plan to attend will be able to tell you about the requirements for licensure and the courses you will need to meet those requirements.

Most graduate-level art therapy educational programs require specific prerequisites, including courses in psychology and studio art, plus an art portfolio demonstrating competency in drawing, painting, and sculpture. Some programs will want you to have a strong art background, while others may require a minimal level of experience with visual art. While you do not need an undergraduate degree in art therapy, you generally must show evidence of successful paid or volunteer work with people in a community, recreational place, hospital, or mental health setting.

Most graduate-level educational programs in the United States follow standards for art therapy education developed and approved by the AATA. Courses cover the following:

- history and development of the field
- methods and materials
- techniques with children, adults, and families
- art therapy theory and practice with special populations (for example, people with psychiatric or medical problems, developmental delays, or physical disabilities)
- human development, career, and individual, family, and group counseling
- diagnosis and appraisal of mental disorders
- professional ethics and standards of practice
- multicultural issues
- assessment techniques and treatment planning
- research methods in art therapy, counseling, and psychology

A supervised practicum is also required as part of the degree and usually includes your working under supervision of an art therapist at several different settings. For example, within your practicum you might work on the pediatric ward of a hospital, in a mental health clinic with adult psychiatric patients, in a school for children with developmental disabilities, and in a geriatric facility.

Many art therapists go on after graduation to obtain other credentials demonstrating education and professional competence in addition to their master's degree. An art therapist registered (ATR), a credential provided by the Art Therapy Credentials Board (ATCB), is awarded to individuals who successfully complete an approved master's degree in art therapy or a related field and one thousand hours of postgraduate experience in art therapy. There are also board-certified art therapists (ATR-BC), who have completed the requirements for ATR and have passed a certification examination administered by the ATCB. In some states, one can become a licensed professional art therapist (LPAT), a certified professional art therapist (CPAT), or a licensed creative arts therapist (LCAT). In many other states, art therapists can also become licensed as professional counselors (LPC), clinical mental health counselors (LPCC or LMHC), or marriage and family therapists (LMFT).

Again, being licensed may or may not be important, depending on your career goals. For example, I chose to become licensed as a clinical mental health counselor so that I could practice art therapy in medical settings, establish a private practice, and be eligible for reimbursement from insurance and managed-care health plans from patients. In most states, the practice of any type of therapy or mental health counseling requires licensure by the state, and in some circumstances, it may be a violation of the law to practice art therapy without a license or appropriate credentials.

If you are looking for an undergraduate or graduate training program in the United States, the AATA can provide a list of current educational programs. While there are formal art therapy training programs, people take different routes to learning about art therapy and integrating it into their work with people. For example, psychologists, counselors, and social workers may take courses in art therapy, expressive therapy, or creative arts therapies in order to learn more about how to use art in treating their clients. Some schools offer certificate programs for people with related master's degrees (such as psychology, social work, counseling, special education, or art), which include courses and practicum experiences similar to those within an art therapy master's program. If you wish to become an ATR or ATR-BC, it is important that you contact the AATA and ATCB to determine if the educational program you wish to attend will help you eventually qualify for one or both of these credentials.

Lastly, if you live in a country other than the United States, it is important to know that art therapy training varies throughout the world. What I have included in the following brief section describes art therapy training and requirements for credentials within the United States. Because training is substantially different in other countries, resources for international art therapy associations are included in the subsequent section.

Art Therapy Organizations in the United States

The **American Art Therapy Association (AATA)** is the national organization of art therapists in the United States; it also has members in more than thirty other countries throughout the world. The AATA is dedicated to encouraging high standards for education and practice in the field and disseminating public information. The organization holds an annual conference and publishes books and monographs on art therapy, proceedings from annual conferences, and a quarterly journal, *Art Therapy: Journal of the American Art Therapy Association*.

arttherapy.org
E-mail: info@arttherapy.org
5999 Stevenson Avenue
Alexandria, VA 22304
888-290-0878

The AATA originally set standards for credentials for art therapists in the United States. However, in 1991, a separate credentials board, the **Art Therapy Credentials Board (ATCB)**, was established. If you are interested in obtaining an application for registration or certification as an art therapist, this is the board to contact.

atcb.org
E-mail: atcb@nbcc.org
3 Terrace Way, Suite B
Greensboro, NC 27403-3660
877-213-2822

International Organizations

The **British Association of Art Therapists (BAAT)** is the professional organization for art therapists in the United Kingdom and has its own code of ethics of professional practice. Comprising twenty regional groups, a European and an international section, the BAAT maintains a comprehensive directory of qualified art therapists and works to promote art therapy in the United Kingdom.

baat.org/index.html
E-mail: info@baat.org
24-27 White Lion Street
London, England N1 9PD
020 7686 4216; fax: 020 7837 7945

The **International Networking Group for Art Therapists (INGAT)** is a worldwide, Internet-based group of art therapists representing approximately eighty countries. The group can assist you if you are looking for information on the practice of art therapy outside the United States.

emporia.edu/ingat

Other Organizations

The **National Coalition of Creative Arts Therapies Associations (NCCATA)** is an umbrella coalition of national art therapy, music therapy, dance therapy, drama therapy, and poetry therapy organizations. It can refer you to other art therapy associations throughout the United States, and its website serves as a link to major art therapy organizations.

nccata.org
c/o AMTA
8455 Colesville Road, Suite 1000
Silver Spring, MD 20910

The **European Consortium for Arts Therapies Education (ECArTE)** is a consortium of universities and other institutions of higher education. Its primary purpose is to represent and encourage the development of the arts therapies at a European level—in particular, the courses offering nationally validated and professionally recognized training for arts therapists. (The arts therapies include art therapy, dance therapy, drama therapy, and music therapy.)

uni-muenster.de/ecarte
E-mail: members@ecarte.info

The **International Expressive Arts Therapy Association (IEATA)** serves as a nonprofit professional organization to support and provide a national and international exchange within the expressive arts field for artists, educators, and therapists.

ieata.org
E-mail: ieata@ieata.org
P.O. Box 320399
San Francisco, CA 94132-0399
415-522-8359

The **Arts in Therapy International Alliance (AITIA)**—therapeutic arts in all shapes and sizes: projects, finds, research, resources, thinking, learning, growth oriented expression.

arts-in-therapy.blogspot.com

The mission of the **American Music Therapy Association (AMTA)** is to advance public awareness of the benefits of music therapy and increase access to quality music therapy services throughout the United States and the rest of the world.

musictherapy.org
E-mail: info@musictherapy.org
8455 Colesville Road, Suite 1000
Silver Spring, MD 20910
301-589-3300; fax: 301-589-5175

Founded in 1966, the **American Dance Therapy Association (ADTA)** works to establish and maintain high standards of professional education and competence in the field of dance or movement therapy. The ADTA publishes the *ADTA Newsletter*, the *American Journal of Dance Therapy*, monographs, bibliographies, and conference proceedings.

adta.org
E-mail: info@adta.org
2000 Century Plaza, Suite 108
10632 Little Patuxent Parkway
Columbia, MD 21044
410-997-4040; fax: 410-997-4048

The **National Association for Drama Therapy (NADT)** establishes and upholds standards of professional competence and ethics among drama therapists, develops criteria for training and registration, and promotes the profession of drama therapy through information and advocacy.

nadt.org
15 Post Side Lane
Pittsford, NY 14534
585-381-5618; fax: 585-383-1474

The **American Society of Group Psychotherapy and Psychodrama (ASGPP)** was founded in 1942 by J. L. Moreno, M.D. (1889–1974). The organization continues to be a source for ongoing developments in group psychotherapy, psychodrama, and sociometry.

asgpp.org
E-mail: asgpp@asgpp.org
301 N. Harrison Street, Suite 508
Princeton, NJ 08540
609-452-1339; fax: 609-936-1659

The **National Association for Poetry Therapy (NAPT)** supports the work of poetry therapists in mental health, medical, geriatric, therapeutic, educational, and community settings.

poetrytherapy.org
E-mail: info@poetrytherapy.org
525 SW 5th Street, Suite A
Des Moines, IA 50309-4501
866-844-NAPT or 515-282-8192; fax: 515-282-9117

Related Websites and Resources

PapaInk, the International Children's Art Archive, has an ongoing online exhibition of works by young artists. It is dedicated to the archiving of historically significant children's art collections and the building of communities that support children's creative endeavors.

papaink.org

Hospital Audiences, Inc. (HAI) is a not-for-profit organization founded in 1969 to provide access to the arts to culturally isolated New Yorkers, including people with mental and physical disabilities, mentally retarded/developmentally disabled persons, bed-confined/wheelchair-users, visually and hearing-impaired individuals, the homeless, the frail elderly, youth at risk, participants in substance abuse programs, persons with HIV/AIDS, and individuals in correctional facilities.

hospaud.org
E-mail: hai@hospaud.org
548 Broadway, 3rd Floor
New York, NY 10012
212-575-7676; fax: 212-575-7669

The **Arts and Healing Network (AHN)** site was created in 1997 as an online resource for people interested in the healing potential of art. At the beginning of each month, it publishes a new issue of its online newsletter, *AHN News*, which includes books reviews, links, and interviews with leaders in the field of art and healing.

artheals.org

The **Foundation for Hospital Art** is dedicated to improving hospital environments with colorful paintings, wall murals, and ceiling tiles. Participants paint predrawn, color-coded designs at PaintFests held in a variety of settings around the world. The artwork is touched up and then donated to needy hospitals on behalf of the sponsor.

hospitalart.com
120 Stonemist Court
Roswell, GA 30076
770-645-1717; fax: 770-645-1720

Survivors Art Foundation (SAF) is dedicated to encouraging healing through the arts and empowering trauma survivors with effective expressive outlets via an Internet art gallery, outreach programs, national exhibitions, publications, and development of employment skills.

survivorsartfoundation.org
E-mail: safe@survivorsartfoundation.org
P.O. Box 383
Westhampton, NY 11977

The **Center for Therapy Through the Arts** is a provider of customized art therapy services for special needs populations, art therapy professionals, and individuals and groups seeking unique art therapy programs.

therapythruart.org
E-mail: therapythruart@yahoo.com
12200 Fairhill Road
Cleveland, OH 44120
216-791-9303

A nonprofit youth arts organization, **Raw Art Works (RAW)**, founded in 1988, provides young people with innovative ways to engage in art making that can and does transform their lives.

rawart.org
E-mail: mail@rawart.org
37 Central Square
Lynn, MA 01901
781-593-5515

OFFCenter Community Arts Project is a community art space located in the heart of Albuquerque, New Mexico. The center is home to a studio, a gallery, and a sales shop. Anyone in the community is welcome to come to OFFCenter to make and buy art. Artists of low income are especially encouraged to make art in the studio, sell their work in the sales shop, and submit their work for display in the gallery. Individuals, families, and groups participate in a wide variety of both casual open studios and organized activities.

offcenterarts.org
E-mail: info@offcenterarts.org
808 Park Avenue SW
Albuquerque, NM 87102
505-247-1172

The **Open Studio Project (OSP)** is dedicated to art making and providing service to the public through workshops, open studio art-making opportunities, and special events.

openstudioproject.org
903 Sherman Avenue
Evanston, IL 60202
847-475-0390

The **Creative Growth Art Center** serves adult artists who are physically, mentally, and developmentally disabled. The center provides stimulating environments for instruction and exhibition.

creativegrowth.org
355 Twenty-Fourth Street
Oakland, CA 94612
510-836-2340

The **American Institute of Medical Education (AIMED)** provides information, lectures, and conferences on creativity and artists and holds Creativity and Madness conferences throughout the world.

aimed.com

The **Prinzhorn Collection** site provides information on Hans Prinzhorn and art contained in the collection. Prinzhorn was one of the first authorities on psychiatric illness and artistic expression.

prinzhorn.uni-hd.de/index_eng.shtml

Journals and Periodicals

The following professional art therapy journals are available at many university libraries or by subscription.

The Arts in Psychotherapy
Elsevier Science
660 White Plains Road
Tarrytown, NY 10591-5153

Art Therapy: Journal of the American Art Therapy Association
arttherapy.org
5999 Stevenson Avenue
Alexandria, VA 22304
888-290-0878

Books on Art Therapy and Related Subjects

Cane, Florence. *The Artist in Each of Us*. Craftsbury Common, VT: Art Therapy Publications, 1983.

Case, Caroline, and Tessa Dalley, eds. *The Handbook of Art Therapy*. London: Tavistock, 1992.

Cohen, Barry, and Carol Thayer. *Telling Without Talking: Art as a Window into the World of Multiple Personality*. New York: Norton, 1995.

Furth, Gregg M. *The Secret World of Drawings*. Boston: Sigo, 1988.

Gladding, Samuel T. *Counseling as an Art: The Creative Arts in Counseling*, 3rd ed. Alexandria, VA: American Counseling Association, 2004.

Junge, Maxine, and Paige Asawa. *A History of Art Therapy in the United States*. Mundelein, IL: AATA, Inc., 1994.

Kaye, Charles, and Tony Blee, eds. *The Arts in Health Care: A Palette of Possibilities*. London: Jessica Kingsley, 1996.

Kellogg, Joan. *Mandala: Path of Beauty*, 3rd ed. Clearwater, FL: ATMA, 2002.

Kellogg, Rhoda. *Analyzing Children's Art*. Palo Alto, CA: Mayfield, 1970.

Klorer, Patricia. *Expressive Therapy with Troubled Children*. Northvale, NJ: Jason Aronson, 2000.

Knill, Paolo, Helen Barba, and Margot Fuchs. *Minstrels of the Soul: Intermodal Expressive Therapy*. Toronto: Palmerston Press, 1995.

Kramer, Edith. *Art as Therapy with Children*, 2nd ed. Chicago: Magnolia, 1993.

Kwiatkowska, Hanna Yaxa. *Family Therapy and Evaluation Through Art*. Springfield, IL: Charles C. Thomas, 1978.

Landgarten, Helen B. *Clinical Art Therapy*. New York: Brunner/Mazel, 1981.

Lynn, Darcy. *Myself Resolved*. Vienna, VA: Strategic Communications, 1996.

MacGregor, John M. *The Discovery of the Art of the Insane*. Princeton, NJ: Princeton University Press, 1989.

Malchiodi, Cathy A. *Breaking the Silence: Art Therapy with Children from Violent Homes*. Bristol, PA: Brunner/Mazel, 1997.

———. *Understanding Children's Drawings*. New York: Guilford, 1998.

Malchiodi, Cathy A., ed. *Expressive Therapies*. New York: Guilford, 2005.

———. *Handbook of Art Therapy*. New York: Guilford, 2003.

———. *Medical Art Therapy with Children*. London: Jessica Kingsley, 1998.

McNiff, Shaun. *Art as Medicine*. Boston: Shambhala, 1994.

———. *Art Heals*. Boston: Shambhala, 2005.

———. *The Arts in Psychotherapy*. Springfield, IL: Charles C. Thomas, 1981.

Moon, Bruce. *Existential Art Therapy*, 2nd ed. Springfield, IL: Charles C. Thomas, 1995.

Naumburg, Margaret. *Dynamically Oriented Art Therapy*. Chicago: Magnolia, 1993 (originally published in 1966).

Orleman, Jane. *Telling Secrets: An Artist's Journey Through Childhood Trauma*. Washington, DC: Child Welfare League of America, 1998.

Oster, Gerald, and Patricia Gould. *Using Drawings in Assessment and Therapy*, 2nd ed. New York: Brunner/Mazel, 2004.

Panter, Barry, ed. *Creativity and Madness: Psychological Studies of Art and Artists*. Burbank, CA: AIMED Press, 1995.

Riley, Shirley. *Contemporary Art Therapy with Adolescents*. London: Jessica Kingsley, 1999.

———. *Group Process Made Visible*. New York: Brunner-Routledge, 2001.

Riley, Shirley, and Cathy A. Malchiodi. *Integrative Approaches to Family Art Therapy*. Chicago: Magnolia, 1994.

Robbins, Arthur. *The Artist as Therapist*. New York: Human Sciences Press, 1987.

Rogers, Natalie. *The Creative Connection: Expressive Arts as Healing*. Palo Alto, CA: Science & Behavior Books, 1993.

Rubin, Judith. *Approaches to Art Therapy*, 2nd ed. New York: Brunner/Mazel, 2001.

———. *Art Therapy: An Introduction*. Bristol, PA: Brunner/Mazel, 1998.

Safran, Diane. *Art Therapy and ADHD: Diagnostic and Therapeutic Approaches*. London: Jessica Kingsley, 2002.

Simon, Rita. *Symbolic Images in Art as Therapy*. New York: Routledge, 1997.

Spencer, Linda B. *Heal Abuse and Trauma Through Art*. Springfield, IL: Charles C. Thomas, 1997.

Ulman, Elinor, and Penny Dachinger, eds. *Art Therapy in Theory and Practice*. Chicago: Magnolia, 1996 (originally published in 1975).

Wadeson, Harriet. *Advances in Art Therapy*. New York: Wiley, 1989.

———. *Art Psychotherapy*. New York: Wiley, 1980.

Waller, Diane. *Group Interactive Art Therapy*. New York: Routledge, 1993.

Books to Stimulate Art Making

Allen, Pat B. *Art Is a Way of Knowing*. Boston: Shambhala, 1995.

Beam, Mary Todd. *Celebrate Your Creative Self*. Cincinnati, OH: North Light Books, 2001.

Harrison, Holly, and Paula Grasdal. *Collage for the Soul*. Gloucester, MA: Rockport, 2003.

London, Peter. *No More Secondhand Art*. Boston: Shambhala, 1989.

Malchiodi, Cathy A. *The Soul's Palette: Drawing on Art's Transformative Powers for Health and Well-Being*. Boston: Shambhala, 2002.

McNiff, Shaun. *Trust the Process*. Boston: Shambhala, 1998.

Perrella, Lynne. *Artists, Journals, and Sketchbooks*. Gloucester, MA: Quarry, 2004.

Art Supplies

The following companies have mail-order catalogs from which you can order the art supplies described in this book.

NASCO Arts & Crafts
enasco.com/artsandcrafts
901 Janesville Avenue
P.O. Box 901
Fort Atkinson, WI 53538-0901
800-558-9595

Pearl Art Supplies
pearlpaint.com
308 Canal Street
New York, NY 10013
800-451-7327

Sax Arts & Crafts
saxarts.com
2727 S. Moorland Road
New Berlin, WI 53151
800-558-6696

Selected References

Chapter 1

Allen, Pat B. *Art Is a Way of Knowing*. Boston: Shambhala, 1995.

Ault, Robert. *Drawing on the Contours of the Mind*. Self-published manuscript, date unknown.

Dissanayake, Ellen. *What Is Art For?* Seattle: University of Washington Press, 1989.

Freud, Sigmund. "The Ego and the Id." In J. Strachey, ed., *The Complete Psychological Works of Sigmund Freud. XIX*. London: Hogarth, 1923.

Gendlin, Eugene. *Focusing-Oriented Psychotherapy*. New York: Guilford Publications, 1998.

Gross, J., and H. Haynes. "Drawing Facilitates Children's Verbal Reports of Emotionally-Laden Events." *Journal of Experimental Psychology* 4: 163–179, 1998.

Jung, Carl Gustav, Marie-Louise Von Franz, and Joseph Henderson. *Man and His Symbols*. New York: Doubleday, 1968.

Kaplan, Frances. *Art, Science, and Art Therapy*. London: Jessica Kingsley, 2000.

Lambert, Don. *The Life and Art of Elizabeth "Grandma" Layton*. Topeka, KS: WRS, 1995.

London, Peter. *No More Secondhand Art*. Boston: Shambhala, 1989.

Malchiodi, Cathy A. *Breaking the Silence: Art Therapy with Children from Violent Homes*. Bristol, PA: Brunner/Mazel, 1997.

Maslow, Abraham. *Toward a Psychology of Being*, rev. ed. New York: John Wiley & Sons, 1968.

May, Rollo. *My Quest for Beauty*. Dallas: Saybrook, 1985.

Moon, Bruce. *Existential Art Therapy*. Springfield, IL: Charles C. Thomas, 1995.

Rubin, Judith. *Art Therapy: An Introduction*. Philadelphia: Brunner/Mazel, 1998.

Wadeson, Harriet. *Art Psychotherapy*. New York: John Wiley & Sons, 1980.

Chapter 2

Adamson, Edward. *Art as Healing*. London: Conventure, 1990.

Gablik, Suzi. *The Re-enchantment of Art*. New York: Thames & Hudson, 1991.

Gladding, Samuel. *Counseling as an Art: The Creative Arts in Counseling*, 3rd ed. Alexandria, VA: American Counseling Association, 2004.

Goodenough, Florence. *Measurement of Intelligence by Drawings*. New York: Harcourt, Brace, & World, 1926.

Hill, Adrian. *Art Versus Illness*. London: Allen & Unwin, 1945.

———. *Painting Out Illness*. London: Williams & Northgate, 1951.

Jamison, Kay Redfield. *Touched with Fire*. New York: Free Press, 1993.

Jung, Carl Gustav. *Mandala Symbolism*. Princeton, NJ: Princeton University Press, 1959.

Knill, Paolo, Helen Barba, and Margo Fuchs. *Minstrels of the Soul: Intermodal Expressive Therapy*. Toronto: Palmiston Press, 1995.

Kramer, Edith. *Art as Therapy with Children*, 2nd ed. Chicago: Magnolia, 1993.

Kwiatkowska, Hanna Yaxa. *Family Therapy and Evaluation Through Art*. Springfield, IL: Charles C. Thomas, 1978.

MacGregor, John. *The Discovery of the Art of the Insane*. Princeton, NJ: Princeton University Press, 1989.

———. "Paul-Max Simon: The Father of Art and Psychiatry." *Art Therapy: Journal of the American Art Therapy Association* 1 (1): 8–20, 1983.

Malchiodi, Cathy A., ed. *Handbook of Art Therapy*. New York: Guilford Publications, 2003.

May, Rollo. *The Courage to Create*. New York: Norton, 1975.

McNiff, Shaun. *The Arts and Psychotherapy*. Springfield, IL: Charles C. Thomas, 1981.

National Center for Complementary and Alternative Medicine. "Major Domains of Complementary and Alternative Medicine." Available at http://nih.gov/fcp/classify/, 2005.

Naumburg, Margaret. *An Introduction to Art Therapy*. New York: Teachers College Press, 1973.

Panter, Michael. *Creativity and Madness: Psychological Studies of Art and Artists*. Burbank, CA: AIMED Press, 1995.

Prinzhorn, Hans. *Artistry of the Mentally Ill*. New York: Springer-Verlag, 1972 (originally published in 1922).

Rhyne, Janie. *The Gestalt Art Experience*, 2nd ed. Chicago: Magnolia, 1995.

Salina Art Center. *Beyond the Drawing Room: The Art of Mary Huntoon*. Salina, KS: Salina Art Center, 1994.

Siegel, Bernie. *Love, Medicine, and Miracles*. New York: Harper & Row, 1986.

Spoerri, Elka, ed. *Adolph Wolfli: Draftsman, Writer, Poet, Composer*. Ithaca, NY: Cornell University Press, 1997.

Ulman, Elinor, and Peggy Dachinger. *Art Therapy in Theory and Practice*. Chicago: Magnolia, 1996.

Wadeson, H. *Art Psychotherapy*. New York: John Wiley & Sons, 1980.

Chapter 3

Allen, Pat B. *Art Is a Way of Knowing*. Boston: Shambhala, 1995.

Erikson, Erik. *Toys and Reasons*. New York: Norton, 1977.

Gardner, Howard. *Artful Scribbles*. New York: Basic Books, 1980.

Jung, Carl Gustav. *Psychological Types*. London: Kegan Paul, 1923.

Malchiodi, Cathy A. *Understanding Children's Drawings*. New York: The Guilford Press, 1998.

Nachmanovitch, Stephen. *Free Play*. Los Angeles: Jeremy Tarcher, 1990.

Chapter 4

American Art Therapy Association Mission Statement. Mundelein, IL: AATA, Inc., 1996.

Cohen, Gene. *The Creative Age: Awakening Human Potential in the Second Half of Life*. New York: HarperCollins, 2000.

Czikszentmihalyi, Mihaly. *Flow: The Psychology of Optimal Experience*. New York: Harper & Row, 1990.

Freud, Sigmund. *On Creativity and the Unconscious*. New York: Harper & Row, 1953.

Gardner, Howard. *Creating Minds*. New York: Basic Books, 1993.

Jung, Carl Gustav. *Memories, Dreams, Reflections*. New York: Pantheon, 1961.

Lusebrink, Vija. *Imagery and Visual Expression in Therapy*. New York: Plenum Press.

Malchiodi, Cathy A. *The Soul's Palette: Drawing on Art's Transformative Powers for Health and Well-Being*. Boston: Shambhala, 2002.

May, Rollo. *The Courage to Create*. New York: Norton, 1975.

———. *My Quest for Beauty*. Dallas: Saybrook, 1985.

McNiff, Shaun. *Trust the Process*. Boston: Shambhala, 1998.

Rogers, Carl. *On Becoming a Person*. Boston: Houghton Mifflin, 1961.

Chapter 5

Capacchione, Lucia. *The Creative Journal*. Chicago: Swallow, 1979.

Erikson, Joan. *Wisdom and the Senses: The Way of Creativity*. New York: Norton, 1988.

Landgarten, Helen. *Family Art Psychotherapy*. New York: Brunner/Mazel, 1987.

Chapter 6

Arguelles, José, and Miriam Arguelles. *Mandala*. Boston: Shambhala, 1995.

Cane, Florence. *The Artist in Each of Us*, rev. ed. Craftsbury Common, VT: Art Therapy Publications, 1983.

Capacchione, Lucia. *The Power of the Other Hand*. Hollywood, CA: Newcastle, 1988.

Jung, Carl Gustav. *Mandala Symbolism*. Princeton, NJ: Princeton University Press, 1959.

Kellogg, Joan. *Mandala: Path of Beauty*. Lightfoot, VA: MARI, 1991.

Naumburg, Margaret. *Dynamically Oriented Art Therapy*. New York: Grune & Stratton, 1966.

Virshup, Evelyn. *Right Brain People in a Left Brain World*. Los Angeles: Art Therapy West, 1979.

Winnicott, Donald. *Therapeutic Consultations in Child Psychiatry*. New York: Basic Books, 1971.

Chapter 7

Arnheim, Rudolph. *To the Rescue of Art: Twenty-six Essays*. Berkeley, CA: University of California, 1992.

Gross, J., and H. Haynes. "Drawing Facilitates Children's Verbal Reports of Emotionally-Laden Events." *Journal of Experimental Psychology* 4: 163–179, 1998.

Jones, John Goff. "Art Therapy with a Community of Survivors." *Art Therapy: Journal of the American Art Therapy Association* 14 (2): 89–94, 1997.

Jung, Carl Gustav. *Memories, Dreams, Reflections*. New York: Pantheon, 1961.

Kübler-Ross, Elisabeth. *Living with Death and Dying*. New York: MacMillan, 1981.

Levine, Peter. *Healing Trauma*. Boulder, CO: Sounds True, Inc., 2005.

Malchiodi, Cathy A. "Art and Loss." *Art Therapy: Journal of the American Art Therapy Association* 9 (3), 1992.

———. "Art Therapy and the Brain." In Cathy A. Malchiodi (ed.), *Handbook of Art Therapy* (pp. 16–24). New York: Guilford Publications, 2003.

———. *Breaking the Silence: Art Therapy with Children from Violent Homes*. Bristol, PA: Brunner/Mazel, 1997.

McNiff, Shaun. *Art as Medicine*. Boston: Shambhala, 1994.

Orleman, Jane. "Looking In—Looking Out: An Artist's Journey Through Child Sexual Abuse." *Art Therapy: Journal of the American Art Therapy Association* 11 (1): 54–56, 1994.

———. *Telling Secrets: An Artist's Journey Through Childhood Trauma*. Washington, DC: Child Welfare League of America, 1998.

Van der Kolk, Bessel, Alexander McFarlane, and Lars Weisaeth. *Traumatic Stress: The Effects of Overwhelming Experience on Mind, Body, and Society*. New York: Guilford Publications, 1996.

Chapter 8

Achterburg, Jeanne. *Imagery in Healing*. New York: Random House, 1985.

Achterburg, Jeanne, Barbara Dossey, and Leslie Kolkenmeier. *Rituals of Healing: Using Imagery for Health & Wellness*. New York: Bantam/Doubleday, 1994.

Bach, Susan. *Life Paints Its Own Span*. Zurich: Daimon, 1990.

Barasch, Marc Ian. *Healing Dreams: Exploring Dreams That Can Transform Your Life*. New York: Riverhead, 2000.

Berstein, Jane. "Art & Endometriosis." *Art Therapy: Journal of the American Art Therapy Association* 12 (1), 1995.

Cohen, Gene. *The Creative Age: Awakening Human Potential in the Second Half of Life*. New York: HarperCollins, 2000.

Council, Tracy. "Medical Art Therapy with Pediatric Patients." In Cathy A. Malchiodi (ed.), *Handbook of Art Therapy* (pp. 207–219). New York: Guilford Publications, 2003.

Gabriels, Robin. "Art Therapy Assessment of Coping Styles in Severe Asthmatics." *Art Therapy: Journal of the American Art Therapy Association* 5 (2), 1988.

Garfield, Patricia. *The Healing Power of Dreams*. New York: Fireside, 1991.

Graham-Pole, John. *Illness and the Art of Creative Self-Expression: Stories and Exercises from the Arts for Those with Chronic Illness*. New York: New Harbinger Publications, 2000.

Hill, Adrian. *Art Versus Illness*. London: Allen & Unwin, 1945.

———. *Painting Out Illness*. London: Williams & Northgate, 1951.

Jung, Carl Gustav. *Modern Man in Search of a Soul*. New York: Harcourt Brace Jovanovich, 1955.

Kaye, Charles, and Tony Blee, eds. *The Arts in Health Care: A Palette of Possibilities*. London: Jessica Kingsley, 1996.

Kellogg, Joan. *Mandala: Path of Beauty*. Lightfoot, VA: MARI, 1991.

Lynn, Darcy. *Myself Resolved*. Vienna, VA: Strategic Communications, 1996.

Malchiodi, Cathy A. *The Soul's Palette: Drawing on Art's Transformative Powers for Health and Well-Being*. Boston: Shambhala, 2002.

Monti, Daniel, and Caroline Peterson. "Mindfulness-Based Art Therapy." *Psychiatric Times* 21 (8): 63–66, 2004.

National Center for Complementary and Alternative Medicine. "Major Domains of Complementary and Alternative Medicine." Available at http://nih.gov/fcp/classify/, 2005.

Pennebaker, James. *Opening Up: The Healing Power of Confiding in Others*. New York: The Guilford Press, 1997.

Sacks, Oliver. *Awakenings*. New York: Doubleday, 1973.

Sandblom, Paul. *Creativity and Disease: How Illness Affects Literature, Art and Music*, 8th ed. New York: Marion Boyars Publishers, 1995.

Siegel, Bernie. *Love, Medicine, and Miracles*. New York: Harper & Row, 1986.

———. *Peace, Love, and Healing*. New York: HarperCollins, 1990.

Simonton, Carl O., Stephanie Matthews, and James Creighton. *Getting Well Again*. New York: Bantam, 1992.

Van de Castle, Robert L. *Our Dreaming Mind*. New York: Ballantine, 1994.

Chapter 9

Kwiatkowska, Hanna Yaxa. *Family Therapy and Evaluation Through Art*. Springfield, IL: Charles C. Thomas, 1978.

Landgarten, Helen. *Family Art Psychotherapy*. New York: Brunner/Mazel, 1987.

MacGregor, John. *Dwight Mackintosh: The Boy Who Time Forgot*. Oakland, CA: The Creative Growth Art Center, 1992.

Malchiodi, Cathy A. "Family Art Therapy." *Journal of Creativity and Mental Health* 1 (1): 26–40, 2006.

———. *The Soul's Palette: Drawing on Art's Transformative Powers for Health and Well-Being.* Boston: Shambhala, 2002.

Riley, Shirley. "Couples Art Therapy." In Cathy A. Malchiodi (ed.), *Handbook of Art Therapy* (pp. 387–398). New York: Guilford Publications, 2003.

———. *Group Process Made Visible.* New York: Brunner-Routledge, 2001.

Riley, Shirley, and Cathy A. Malchiodi. *Integrative Approaches to Family Art Therapy.* Chicago: Magnolia, 1994.

Waller, Diane. *Group Interactive Art Therapy.* New York: Routledge, 1993.

Yalom, Irving. *Theory and Practice of Group Psychotherapy.* New York: Basic Books, 1995.

Chapter 10

Breuer, Josef. *Studies in Hysteria.* New York: Basic Books, 1982.

De Shazer, Steven. *Words Were Originally Magic.* New York: Norton, 1994.

Freud, Sigmund, and Neil Hertz. *Writings on Art and Literature.* Palo Alto, CA: Stanford University Press, 1997.

Gantt, Linda, and Carmello Tabone. "The Formal Elements Art Therapy Scale (FEATS)." In Cathy A. Malchiodi (ed.), *Handbook of Art Therapy* (pp. 420–427). New York: Guilford Publications, 2003.

Gil, Eliana. *The Healing Power of Play.* New York: Guilford Publications, 1991.

Gladding, Samuel. *Counseling as an Art: The Creative Arts in Counseling,* 3rd ed. Alexandria, VA: American Counseling Association, 2004.

Jung, Carl Gustav. *Memories, Dreams, Reflections.* New York: Pantheon, 1961.

Kellogg, Joan. *Mandala: Path of Beauty,* 3rd ed. Lightfoot, VA: MARI, 2002.

Knill, Paolo, Helen Barba, and Margo Fuchs. *Minstrels of the Soul: Intermodal Expressive Therapy.* Toronto: Palmerston Press, 1995.

Kramer, Edith. "The Art Therapist's Third Hand: Reflections on Art, Art Therapy, and Society at Large." *American Journal of Art Therapy* 24 (3): 71–86, 1986.

Malchiodi, Cathy A., ed. *Expressive Therapies.* New York: Guilford Publications, 2005.

McNiff, Shaun. *Art as Medicine.* Boston: Shambhala, 1994.

Mills, Anne. "The Diagnostic Drawing Series (DDS)." In Cathy A. Malchiodi (ed.), *Handbook of Art Therapy* (pp. 401–409). New York: Guilford Publications, 2003.

Naumburg, Margaret. *Dynamically Oriented Art Therapy.* New York: Grune & Stratton, 1966.

Oster, Gerald, and Patricia Gould. *Using Drawings in Assessment & Therapy.* New York: Brunner-Routledge, 2004.

Pennebaker, James. *Opening Up: The Healing Power of Confiding in Others.* New York: The Guilford Press, 1997.

Rhyne, Janie. *The Gestalt Art Experience,* 2nd ed. Chicago: Magnolia, 1995.

Riley, Shirley, and Cathy A. Malchiodi. *Integrative Approaches to Family Art Therapy*. Chicago: Magnolia, 1994.

———. "Solution-Focused and Narrative Approaches." In Cathy A. Malchiodi (ed.), *Handbook of Art Therapy* (pp. 82–92). New York: Guilford Publications, 2003.

Rogers, Carl. *On Becoming a Person*. Boston: Houghton Mifflin, 1961.

Rogers, Natalie. *The Creative Connection: Expressive Arts as Healing*. Palo Alto, CA: Science & Behavior Books, 1993.

Rubin, Judith. *Approaches to Art Therapy*. New York: Brunner-Routledge, 2001.

Silver, Rawley. *Aggression and Depression Assessed Through Art*. New York: Brunner-Routledge, 2005.

———. *Three Art Assessments: The Silver Drawing Test (SDT), Draw a Story, and Stimulus Drawings and Techniques*. New York: Brunner-Routledge, 2002.

White, Michael, and David Epston. *Narrative Means to Therapeutic Ends*. New York: Norton, 1990.

Index